I0027176

YOGA, MEDITATION AND SPIRITUAL GROWTH FOR THE AFRICAN AMERICAN COMMUNITY

IF YOU CAN BREATHE
YOU CAN DO YOGA AND FIND
INNER AND OUTER PEACE

The Ultimate Yoga Book
for Beginners and the Young At Heart

YOGA, MEDITATION AND SPIRITUAL GROWTH FOR THE AFRICAN AMERICAN COMMUNITY

IF YOU CAN BREATHE
YOU CAN DO YOGA AND FIND
INNER AND OUTER PEACE

The Ultimate Yoga Book
for Beginners and the Young At Heart

Daya Devi-Doolin

Amber Communications Group, Inc.
New York
Phoenix   Los Angeles

YOGA, MEDITATION AND
SPIRITUAL GROWTH FOR THE
AFRICAN AMERICAN COMMUNITY

IF YOU CAN BREATHE
YOU CAN DO YOGA AND FIND
INNER AND OUTER PEACE

By Daya Devi-Doolin

Published by
Amber Books
An Imprint of Amber Communications Group, Inc.
1334 East Chandler Boulevard, Suite 5-D67
Phoenix, AZ 85048
Amberbk@aol.com
WWW.AMBERBOOKS.COM

Tony Rose, Publisher /Editorial Director
Yvonne Rose, Associate Publisher
Tony Rose, Yvonne Rose, Chris Doolin - Editors
The Printed Page, Interior and Cover Design
Photography: Bob Dominguez

Publisher's Note

The Publisher and Author shall have neither liability nor responsibility to any person or organization with respect to any loss or damage caused or alleged to be caused directly or indirectly by the information contained in this book. The purpose of this book is to educate, entertain and stimulate. This book is sold with the understanding that the Publisher and Author are not involved in offering legal, medical or psychological services. If any assistance is required, the services of a competent professional should be sought. In addition, it is not the purpose of this book to be used in the diagnosis of any medical or psychological condition.

All Rights Reserved, including the right to reproduce the book, or any portion thereof, in any form without prior permission of the Publisher, except for the inclusion of brief quotations in a review. Permission granted by Self Realization Fellowship, to use excerpt from *Metaphysical Meditations by* Paramahansa Yogananda. *(See Bibliography for all addresses).*

Copyright 2014 © by Daya Devi-Doolin and Amber Books
ISBN Number: 978-1-937269-46-3
Library of Congress Cataloging-in-Publication Data

Devi-Doolin, Daya, 1941-
  Yoga, meditation and spiritual growth for the African American community : if you can breathe you can do yoga and find inner and outer peace : the ultimate yoga book for beginners and the young at heart / Daya Devi-Doolin.
     pages cm
  Includes bibliographical references.
  ISBN 978-1-937269-46-3
1. Hatha yoga. 2. African Americans--Health and hygiene. I. Title.
  RA781.7.D488 2014
  613.7'046--dc23

                                  2014017026

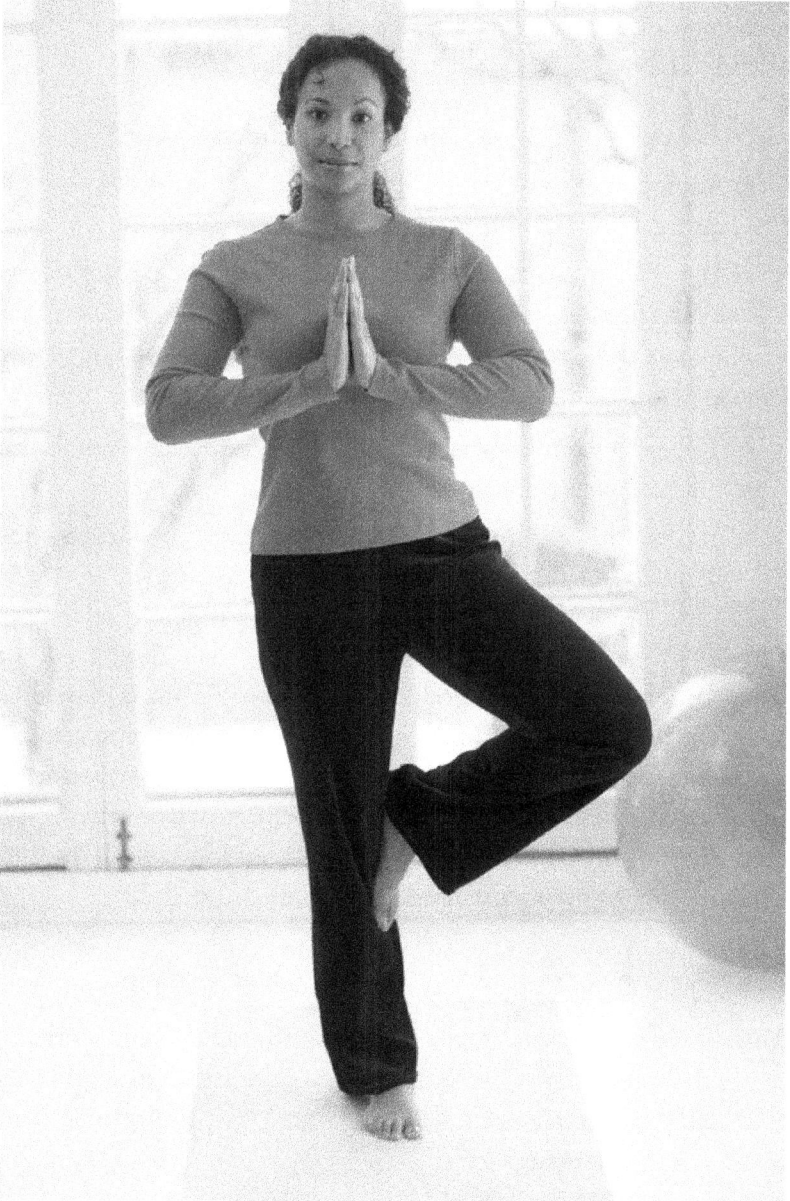

YOGA AND MEDITATION

The Yoga Asanas within this book will, if you practice, help you to burn calories, strengthen the body, mind and soul, offer benefits you cannot even imagine. All you really have to do is KEEP BREATHING!

- The practice of Yoga is loving and limitless.
- Adding yoga to your daily life will bring amazing and positive change's in your life.
- Yoga will arm you, with hope, faith and practical solutions as a healing tool in your life.
- Daya Devi-Doolin has written an excellent, simple and readable book on Hatha Yoga.
- The practice of Yoga is made effortless and easy through the informative in this book.
- You will benefit greatly by applying these teachings to your daily life!

WHY YOGA?

There are millions of people who are suffering from one type of illness or another or debilitation of some kind. They don't realize or haven't been introduced to the beneficial effects of how yoga can help one move beyond limitations and restrictions in order to be free, mobile and excited about life! This book provides hope and direction for a new or a renewed body, mind and spirit.

WHY SHOULD YOU READ THIS BOOK ON YOGA AND MEDITATION?

You should not only read this book, you should take one posture, apply the steps and put the practice into your life. Even if you stay with one posture all week, you will find a vast improvement in your, attitude, body and spirit. You will feel "opened up", cleared and excited about what you have accomplished.

This book can open the door to many wonderful opportunities. A teacher may come, a healing might happen and a peaceful, serene feeling will result. In some instances, asthma has cleared up, lower back pain has disappeared, female problems have healed, arthritic problems in wrists and knees have gone and much more.

HOW DOES THIS BOOK COMPARE TO OTHER BOOKS ON YOGA AND MEDITATION?

The major difference is that this book is for you, the everyday person, the person who works, has a family (or not) and wants to stay stress-free, happy, fulfilled and healthy. This book will lead you, the yoga aspirant, and participant to that place. It has a loveable and knowledgeable approach as if the reader were right in my yoga studio at the Doolin Healing Sanctuary.

The models/photos that are used are real people. The models that are photographed are not size 2 or 8, they are men and women of average shapes, sizes, from various backgrounds and weights.

The one common thing they have is a wish to be healthy, fit, trim, flexible and happy and you can feel that through viewing their practices and postures in a home setting. They are encouraging you to know that you too can do yoga regardless of where you are or how limited you are.

The main idea is that everyone can benefit from yoga and meditation and can start to use it wherever they are in their life.

Yoga is a way of uniting with the Lord. I often talk about six ways to pursue this: Through knowledge (jnana yoga), devotion (bhakti yoga), selfless service (karma yoga), chanting sacred scriptures (mantra yoga), restraint and discipline (raja yoga) and the practice of asanas in Hatha Yoga.

~ Professor Bharat J. Gajjar,
President of the Sivananda Yoga Center of Delaware
and author of several Yoga books and publications.

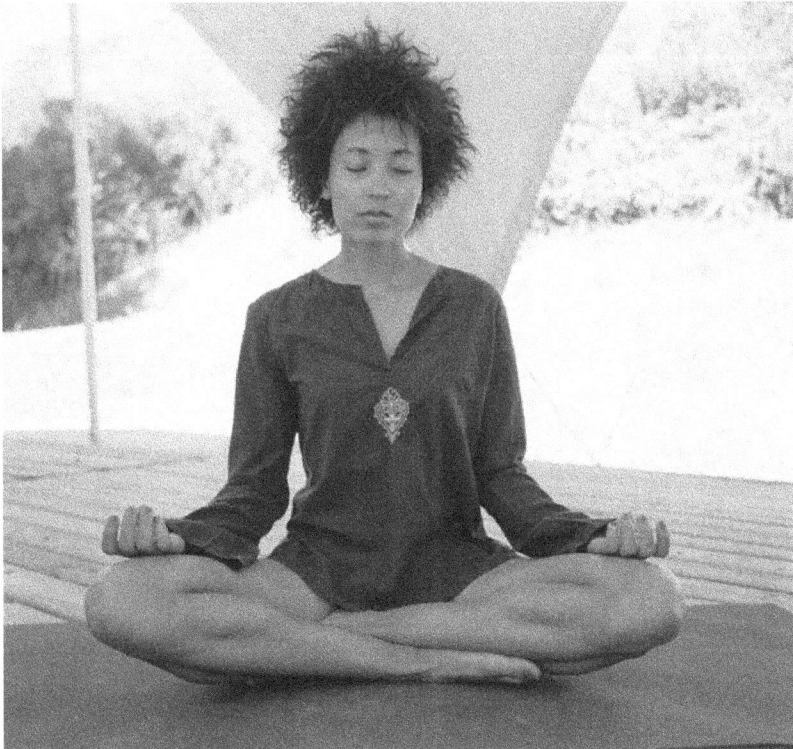

Dedication

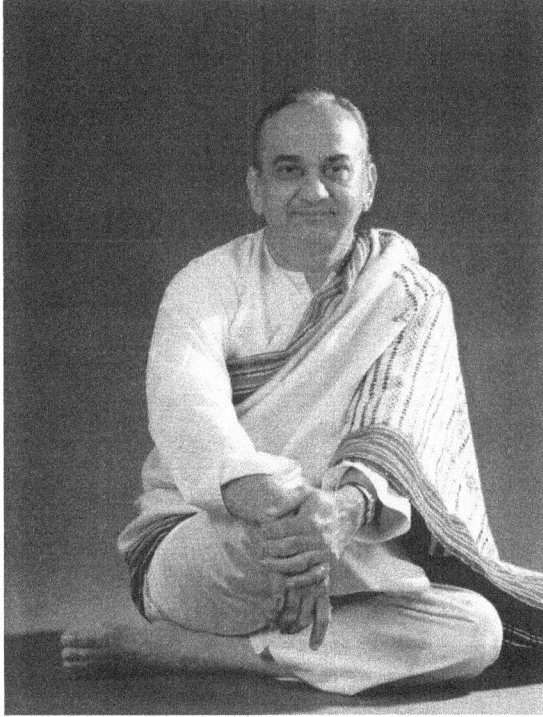

I dedicate this book to my first Yoga Teacher, Professor Yogi Bharat Gajjar and his teacher H.H. Swami Vishnu Devananda.

Acknowledgments

I want to take this opportunity to mention how grateful I am to have had yoga students who wanted to learn true Hatha yoga and the various aspects of it. When I decided to write this book, I asked my students if they would like to be a part of a most wondrous project I was led by the Spirit to be involved in.

The models you see in this book said yes, unequivocally. I want to thank you on this page for your patience, love, devotion and participation to this work.

Shari Niles, Amani Maat Kheru my longtime friend, my husband Chris Doolin, and my sons, Joseph Doolin and Tyler R. Mitchell.

Special thanks to my Publisher and Editor, Tony Rose, for believing in me and my message....

Table of Contents

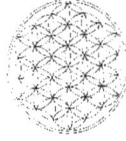

Introduction

Yoga in a Capsule

The Universe honors every thought you have. It honors what you believe in strongly, whether right or wrong for you.
~Daya Devi-Doolin

Yoga in a Capsule

The benefits of Yoga are many and some are below:

1. Deep Relaxation for the body and mind
2. Stress management
3. Maintaining/developing flexibility
4. Building up of muscle strength and length
5. Strengthening of the respiratory and circulatory systems
6. Improved supply of nutrients to all tissues
7. Prevention and alleviation of chronic illnesses (cardiovascular disease, asthma, depression, arthritis and others)
8. Correction of faulty posture and its long-term effects
9. Slowdown of the aging process
10. Enhanced power of concentration
11. Promotion of physical and mental well-being
12. Weight loss and maintenance

I encourage everyone to practice the yoga poses on a regular basis in the quiet of your home and/or in your local yoga studio. Take it slowly with love for yourself and love for the universe. Open your practice with your heart always and give thanks for whatever you can accomplish. Feel good!

The photos I have included are of various students sometimes in the same asanas so you can see the flexibility, mobility and confidence that they have developed. I would like to encourage you to observe how the placement of their feet differs, the spacing between their front and back legs might be wider in some cases, their chests may be raised higher, and lengthening may be longer. Because we are all different, flexibility varies and the time we have practiced varies as well.

We all have our own level of attitude and confidence in ourselves until we can expand into our own perfection. You can reach for the stars and reach to overcome your inner challenges.

I hope your Yoga practice and health are enhanced by the examples in this book, Hatha Yoga classes and Teacher Trainings.

Happy Yoga-ing!

*Namaste', Daya

*Translations: Namaste - *I bow to the Divine Light Within You or I acknowledge the Divine Light (Christ Light) within you. The Divine Light within me blesses the Divine Light within you.*

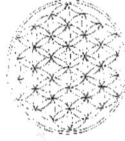

Chapter 1

Getting Started

In helping others to succeed I shall find my own prosperity.
In the welfare of others I shall find my own well-being.
                                                    ~Paramahansa Yogananda

Getting Started – The Foundation of Yoga

I was taught by my favorite Yogi, Professor Yogi Bharat Gajjar, about the Foundation of Yoga, which I have used in my life since I met him. In this book are some of the principles I have learned and used very successfully in my life, and at the same time, helping others to blossom. If you develop virtues like generosity, forgiveness, love, etc., your life will change for the better! He taught that mere yogic kriyas (cleansing) alone would not help. We did self-analysis daily and he suggested that we eradicate our faults and unprofitable habits for a happier life.

Any kind of defects such as selfishness, pride, jealousy and hatred had to no longer be adhered to or tolerated. He taught us to cultivate a compassionate heart.

My name Daya, which was given to me, means compassion. My full name given me during my initiation, means Goddess of

Compassion. I have never been the same after my transformation and initiation into the family of Yoga lineage.

Meeta Gajjar Parker, daughter of my Teacher Bharat Gajjar

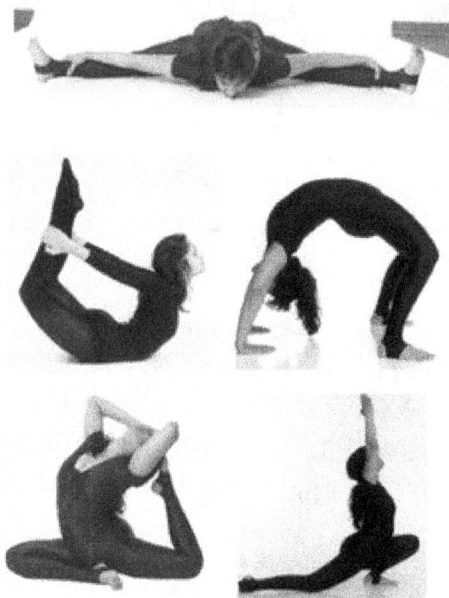

Professor Yogi Bharat Gajjar's Yoga students were taught, paramount to anything, "Purification of the heart because that is of utmost importance." We were taught the yogi aspirant must free himself from lust, anger, greed, hatred, egoism, vanity, attachment, pride and delusion.

This is more difficult than to control the breath or the practice of Nauli (cleansing rolling breathing of the abdomen) or uniting Prana (life-force) and Apana (elimination). "Virtuous qualities such as mercy, tolerance, adaptability, courage, patience, balanced state of mind and cosmic love should be assiduously cultivated." Professor Yogi Bharat Gajjar's message is "With firm faith, practical application, perseverance, simple living, careful attention to even small details and fortitude in trials, you must set foot and proceed on the path of Sadhana." He says, "Yoga is not hidden in caves nor sequestered in the thick Himalayan forests. It is not a mountain herb. God is not a coward to run away from towns, cities and villages. Practice Yoga in your own home. Practice Yoga and preach what you practice. Hatha Yoga ensures sound health, mentally and physically."

- Only in the Silence can Peace Be with you.
- Only in the Silence can you be grateful, full of gratitude and able to calm all those around you with your Light.
- Practice Being in the Silence for 5 minutes a day and breathing.

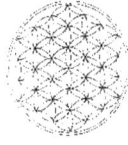

Chapter 2
What is Yoga?

Meditation teaches you how to love or awaken the love that is dormant within you.

~ Yogi Bharat Gajjar

What is Yoga?

Yoga means "union" or "yoke" in Sanskrit. It means the body, mind and spirit become as One, united through the practice of the asanas or postures along with breathing techniques called pranayama and meditation. You can ultimately do yoga by yourself after going to a yoga class for a while, or watching yoga videos to learn more about it visually.

You can get in touch with your body's wisdom through the postures and you know just how far you want to push or challenge yourself. Yoga is so simple, that children, the elderly or anyone who is stiff can easily learn it and benefit from it. Seniors can either use a chair for balance or sit in and practice yoga if they are not quite mobile.

Yoga is an ancient system for personal, physical, mental, emotional and spiritual development. It's good for reducing stress through physical exercises.

It's based on a fundamental principle of East Indian Philosophy that there are five layers or dimensions to human existence:

1. The physical frame.
2. The vital body made of prana (life energy).
3. The mind.
4. The Higher intellect.
5. The abode of bliss where inner peace and union with the Divine occur.

Asanas (postures) can release muscle tension, stretch and tone muscles, lubricate joints, massage internal organs, increase circulation and help in weight control. Yoga postures are comprised of movement sequences performed while standing, sitting, lying down or balancing on your head, shoulders, hands, or bending backward or forward and sideways.

In a structural routine, each pose counterbalances the preceding one by stretching and strengthening. You can investigate your attitude toward yourself and your body. It's a very loving thing, which you can learn to do for yourself and no one else needs to be there. Practitioners report that it has alleviated such conditions as arthritis, scoliosis, back pain, insomnia, chronic fatigue, asthma, heart conditions and much more.

Beginners should look for respect, honesty, carefulness and other qualities they require from a teacher. Trust yourself first. Your gut instincts will tell you if the teacher is pushing you farther than you are ready to go.

A typical yoga practice of postures would include warm-up poses prior to a yoga class or session. Then practice some different standing poses: Triangle pose, hands to feet, standing side stretch pose, stand spread leg forward fold, Warrior pose, tree pose and Sun Salutation. All these poses can be done in a seated fashion as well.

Yoga is a way of uniting with you, since Yoga means "union" or "yoke" in Sanskrit as previously mentioned.

You will be given guided directions with photos that accompany the instructions.

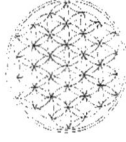

Chapter 3
Yogic Breathing Techniques

Prana, this vital energy is found in all forms of life from mineral to man. Prana is bound in all things having life.
~Swami Vishnu Devananda

Pranayama (Breathing Techniques)

Pranayama is a way to massage the heart and lungs. Prana is an etheric energy that is available to all life forms and is a living force. It gives us better health. It is experienced through yogic breathing, the science of breath control.

One of the techniques that is taught is called Kapalabhati. It's for the lungs and abdomen. It is called a cleansing breath for the nasal passages and respiratory system. Swami Visnu-Devananda, my teacher's Guru says, "In Sanskrit, kapala means skull and bhati means shines." It means it makes the skull shine.

Inhalation is a mild, slow and elongated breath while exhalation is done differently in an important way. The exhalation is done quickly and you do it by forcibly contracting the abdomen with a backward push. This action works upon the diaphragm giving a vigorous push to the lungs, expelling the air from the lungs.

"This is instantly followed by a relaxation of the abdominal muscles, allowing the diaphragm to descend down to the abdominal cavity, pulling with it the lungs. This allows the air to rush in, Kapalabhati. Inhalation and exhalation are done by action of the abdominal muscles and diaphragm." The exhalation is quick, strong and short, while inhalation is passive, slow and longer. Do this for about 36 times, stop for a little while and do another round.

Kapalabhati

Kapalabhati is not technically a pranayama, but one of the Kriyas from Shat Karmas (six cleansing processes in Hatha Yoga), which not only cleanses the skull but also cleans the entire respiratory track. In practice, Kapalabhati is a beginning for pranayama. Guruji Shri Janakinath Brahmachari says, "Before proceeding to the practice of pranayama, everyone should practice Kapalabhati for a few weeks."

The Ha and Tha in Yoga means sun and moon. The sun is represented by the right side of the body and the moon is represented on the left side, which also corresponds to the male and female aspect respectively. The Ha is the Creative Mind and Father and Tha is the Analytic Mind, which is known as Mother.

Technique:

- Sit in any steady and comfortable posture with the back straight, eyes closed and hands on knees.
- Exhale forcefully through both nostrils every time giving an inward stroke at abdomen.
- You could perspire profusely due to the rapid and forceful exhalations. The focus is on active exhalation, whereas inhalation is passive.
- The head and trunk should be kept erect throughout the practice. Practice it continuously according to your capacity,

then stop and allow the mind to relax. Feel the natural cessation of breath.

- This is the automatic suspension of breath for a few seconds or a minute. No urge will be there for breathing during this time. This state is known as Keboli Kumbhaka. Enjoy this state of deep silence and wait for the normal breath to come back.

Initially, you may not be able to do this practice for more than one minute. However, as long as you practice daily with concentration, you will eventually be able to practice many minutes at a stretch, and such daily practice will yield very good results.

Contra-indications: Women during Pregnancy should not practice Kapalabhati. The person suffering from High Blood Pressure or Heart diseases, ulcer or stomach or intestinal diseases, hernia or epilepsy also should not practice.

Benefits

- The practice of Kapalabhati cleanses the entire respiratory system and the nasal passage. It removes spasm in the bronchial tubes and cures asthma.
- It allows carbon dioxide to be eliminated on a large scale, which is not possible through the normal breathing rate of 18 to 20 times per minute for an adult.
- Through regular practice, it also improves the function of the heart, removes migraine pain, sinusitis, and continuous headache, increases stamina and the breathing capacity of lungs.
- It effectively reduces fats around the abdominal area if one practices for a minimum of 20-45 minutes at a stretch.
- Slowly increase time after 30 seconds, more time each day. This is a pure detoxification exercise. Do not eat 1 hour before doing this exercise.

Alternate Nostril – Analoma Viloma

Analoma Viloma (Alternate Nostril Breathing) is another technique I teach to help with concentration of mind and for inner strength. You can sit on floor, a chair, a pillow or mat.

- Thumb is placed on right nostril; ring finger and little finger are used for the left nostril.
- Touch the index and middle finger to your palm of right hand.
- Breathe in through the right nostril, close off both nostrils and allow the breath to flow to lungs.
- Exhale by removing the little finger and ring finger away from the left nostril.
- Breathe in through the left nostril, close off with little finger and ring finger and hold nostrils closed.

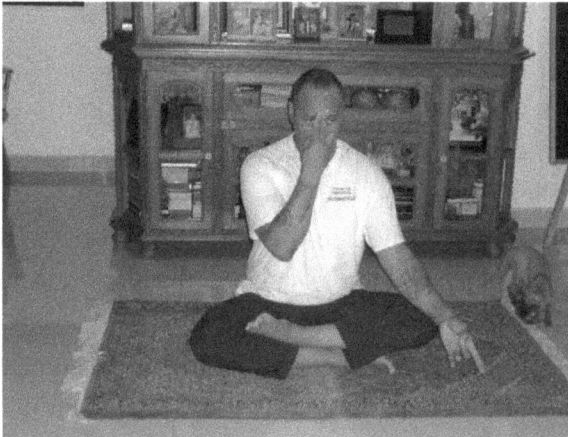

- Allow the intake to flow through you. Breathe in through the right nostril when you have to inhale.
- My yoga teacher taught us to breathe in to the count of 2, hold for the count of 8, exhale to the count of 4. You can double it at any time when you get the hang of it as in inhale to the count of 4, close both nostrils and hold to the count of 16 and exhale to the count of 8. The first technique is just to get you acclimated to the process. Do several rounds of

the technique. I was also taught to chant OM in the mind during the breathing techniques. OM is the Sanskrit word meaning God or Universal Mind.

- He taught us when you or someone gets angry, becomes stressful, fearful, comes in contact with negative or sick people, etc. they will lose prana. You gain prana by positive thinking and living and surrendering to the Holy Spirit.

Practice all pranayama exercises slowly so you won't experience dizziness. You don't have to be afraid because breathing builds lung power, energy for the cells and heart. The breath is known as the Temple of Health, so include it in your daily practice. Make it a new way of living stress-free.

Benefits of Anuloma Viloma

This breathing technique produces greater functioning of both sides of the brain. It leads to a balance between a person's creative side and logical thinking. It calms the mind.

Ujjayi Breathing

Ujjayi means sound breathing. It improves concentration in the physical practice. Sit comfortably cross-legged or in lotus position. The spine is straight. Open your mouth and make the sound you'd make if you were fogging up your glasses to clean them. Do this inhale 2-3 times to get an idea of the sound of making the glasses fogged. The sound happens on the exhale. Now half-way through the inhale, close your mouth and feel and hear the same sound as you breathe in through your nose. It sounds like the Darth Vader sound. It is sometimes called the ocean breath. Hear that sound through your Ujjayi breathing. The tongue is relaxed. Breath is moving in through the throat. Exhaling, you assist the body to release the breath and get rid of excess toxins. Keep your awareness on the flow of your breath and tune into your body and into the world. Continued practice raises your level of consciousness.

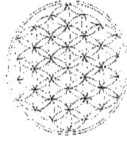

Chapter 4

Yoga Styles

When you become free that means you are detached and you can concentrate on God, which is most difficult to do because detaching from the body and senses is very difficult.
~ Yogi Bharat Gajjar

Yoga Styles

Hatha Yoga is a term that basically means physical types of yoga. It's a gentle style of Yoga (poses or asanas). There are yoga basics such as introduction to yoga, types of yoga and the benefits of yoga. You receive tips for a great yoga practice. There are warm-up poses for all styles of yoga. You are introduced to Yoga and Breathing, table poses, back bends, side bends, standing poses, standing forward bends, seated poses and standing balancing poses. Poses are held for a short period of time and as you advance you learn to transition from one pose to another.

Anusara Yoga is about opening up to Grace with the postures, opening your heart and allowing the breath to flow through; strengthening your core, your muscles and bones and allowing joy to enter. To paraphrase a quote from the founder, "Anusara Yoga is a branch of yoga in the world. This uplifting, healthful and energizing yoga style is becoming a most sought after form of yoga training among professionals. The principles, practices and philosophy of Anusara Yoga are transformative and impact not only your yoga practice, but every aspect of your life!"

Ashtanga is fast paced and kind of a relatively strenuous style of yoga. A series of set poses is taught and performed in the exact same order. It demands constant movement from one pose to the next. Power Yoga stems from Ashtanga, but it does not necessarily keep to the same set of poses. It's based on the flowing movement of Ashtanga.

Vinyasa is another term for various types of classes. It consists of a series of warm-ups that include the breath and movement with the breath. There are a series of poses called Surya Namaskar or Sun Salutation. Each movement is matched with the breath.

Kundalini Yoga is when the focus is on the breath and repetitive movement combined. It frees the energy of the lower body and brings it upwards. It gets rid of toxins by use of the breath (prana) and the movements. Kundalini poses are not held for a long time and the movements are repetitive. It is said to be the most powerful and inclusive of all styles of yoga. It incorporates the techniques and teachings from many different schools of yoga and combines them in such a way as to accelerate the goal of health, well-being, and personal transformation. It consists of exercises or postures (Asanas) with special breathing (Pranayama), hand and finger gestures (Mudras), body locks (Bandhas), and meditation, together or in sequence to create exact, specific effects.

Practitioners state that the results are nothing short of amazing. They've noticed an increase in energy and vitality, flexibility and endurance as well as improved health due to a strengthened immune system.

Iyengar Yoga is based on the teachings of Yogi B.K.S. Iyengar. The poses are held for long periods of time and utilize props to bring the body into alignment. You are taught to get the maximum benefit by being in alignment while practicing.

Bikram Yoga

Bikram method yoga is a twenty-six asana series designed by Bikram Choudhury to scientifically warm and stretch muscles, ligaments and tendons in the proper order. Bikram's twenty-six exercises systematically move fresh, oxygenated blood to one hundred percent of your body, to each organ and fiber, restoring all systems to healthy working order, just as nature intended. Proper weight, muscle tone, vibrant good health, and a sense of well-being will automatically follow. Bikram Yoga is practiced in a heated room about 105 degrees and 40% humidity for 90 minutes. Practitioners will sweat a lot! Don't let this scare you though, Bikram yoga is meant to be done by all. The heat is your friend and will promote flexibility and aid in detoxification.

The method of Yoga I love to teach is called Hatha Yoga. I formulate it to be a gentler style for the age groups I teach, which are generally from 40 to 82 years of age.

In Hatha Yoga, there are stages a beginner works through in attempting the modified boat pose (Navasana).

Modified Boat Pose – Navasana

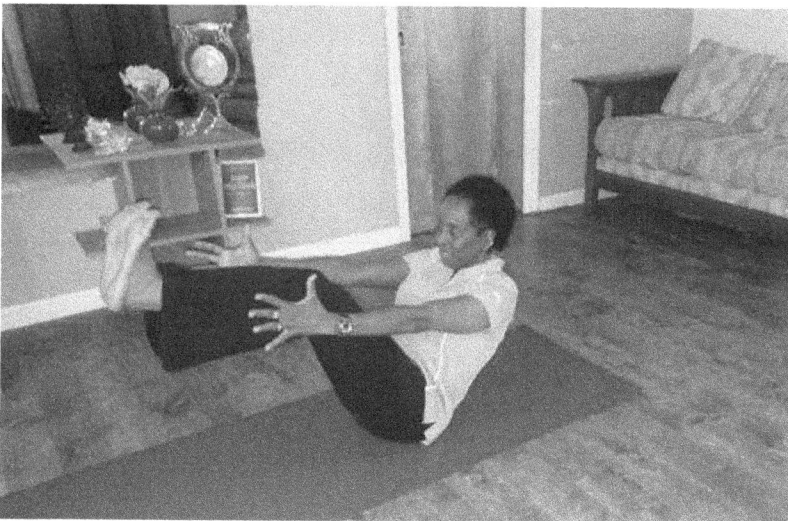

One has to sit and balance on the sitting bones, bend the knees, toes up off the floor. Bring the body into a V-shape by leaning back a bit. Raising the toes to be the same level as the knees, toes are pointing up and heels down. Breathing in, raise the arms along with the knees after you get yourself balanced. Sometimes you can grab your hands under the thighs until you feel balanced, then move the hands away from the knees, and hold them straightened out alongside the knees.

Boat Pose - Navasana

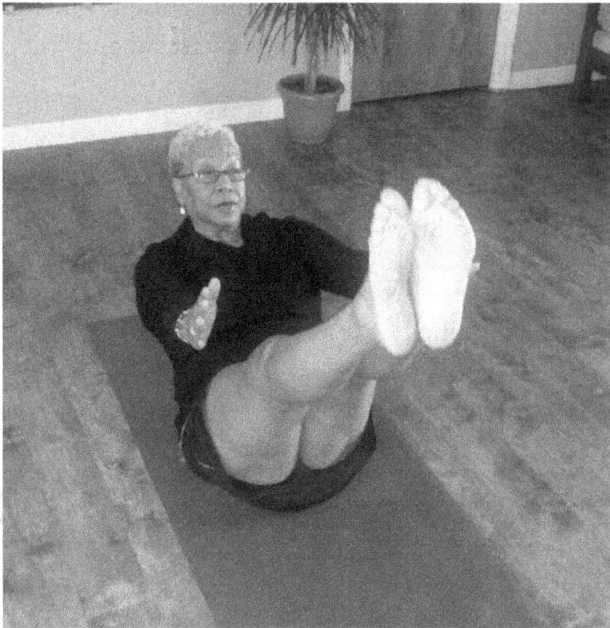

- Prepare by sitting on your sitting bones, bend the knees and make the toes level with the knees; arms outstretched t o the knees, fingers spread open and back straight.
- Vary according to your body flexibility without competition or comparing yourself with another. This will benefit your practice greatly and your body and attitude will flourish.

Forward Bend

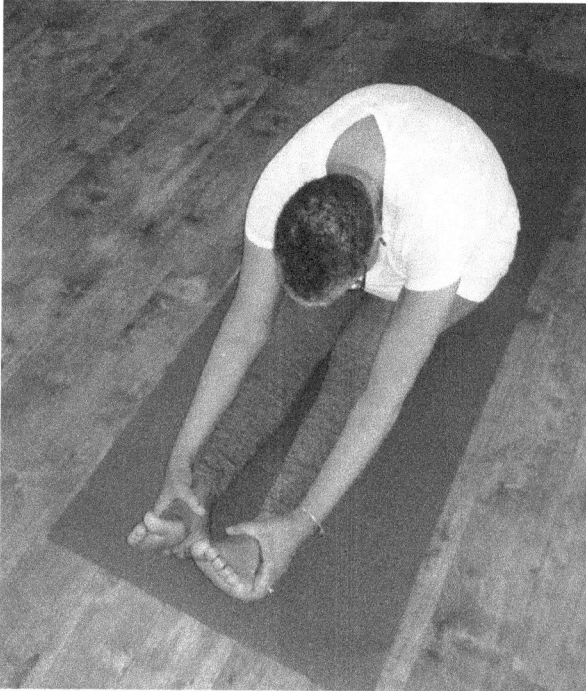

Students start this posture by beginning in Dandasana, a seated pose.

On an inhale, raise your arms up by you ears and fold forward with a straight back, reaching to touch your knees, shins, ankles or toes with your hands as you exhale through nostrils. Then breathe in and out at least five breaths and then relax.

There are also Yoga poses called twists to strengthen the back and poses that are called *supine* poses, in which you are lying on your back. There are backbends, which promote flexibility in the spine, and strengthen your arms, legs and abdomen. There is a *finishing* pose called Corpse Pose or Savasana as a final relaxation at the end of your practice session.

This posture is done lying on your mat. Eyes closed. Feet about 12-inches apart or hips width apart. You palms are up, chest open and relaxed, toes pointed out to sides, and breathing in through the nostrils. This asana can be done before practice, during and after your yoga practice.

Corpse Pose - Savasana

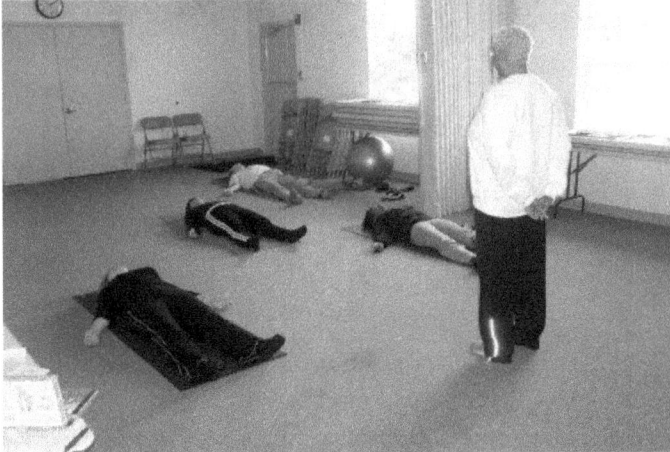

In Savasana, as you breathe in through your nostrils, the abdomen is pushed out by the diaphragm, lungs fill up and the exhale is back up behind the throat and out through the nostrils. Exhaling, the abdomen flattens out and lungs expel waste. Breathing in, softens the face and relaxes the whole body.

Here is a typical comment from one of my students that shows the benefits of Yoga:

> "...My yoga experience has improved my strength, flexibility, anxiety and confidence level. I am no longer experiencing any of the chronic illnesses I had prior to the classes and I have since overcome a long-lasting and painful problem with my back. I have learned, through breathing, how powerful I am and I've been amazed at what I can accomplish physically, spiritually and emotionally."

Yogi Bharat said, "Yoga is a way of uniting with the Lord. I often talk about six ways to pursue this, through:

- Knowledge (jnana yoga)
- Devotion (bhakti yoga)
- Selfless service (karma yoga)
- Chanting sacred scriptures (mantra yoga)
- Restraint and discipline (raja yoga),
- The practice of asanas in Hatha Yoga."

After studying with him for a long time, I thanked Yogi Bharat for being in my life and for the change yoga had made within me.

Little did I know back then, when I started learning to practice Hatha Yoga for myself, that I would be assisting others to be empowered and confident as well.

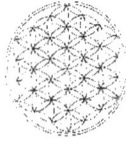

Chapter 5
The Key to Meditating

Meditation is very necessary for man. Meditation is more necessary than sleep. It doesn't matter if you miss sleep even for four days, but it does matter if you are without meditation.

~ Baba Muktananda

The Key to Meditating

The key to meditating is to realize that you are listening to your God Source in the Silence and to focus on the breath. The mind has to follow your command and nothing else when you focus on the inhale and exhale. It cannot focus on doing two things at once, so start by focusing on your breath and then the Silence.

The traditional yoga meditation position (lotus or half lotus) involves sitting cross-legged and breathing in a seated comfortable position on the floor or chair.

If you cannot manipulate sitting cross-legged, try Supta Baddha Konasana. A restorative pose can be done on your back, with soles of feet touching; having the knees bent, sometimes helps, and then a modified cross-legged position works.

Modified Butterfly Pose - Supta Baddha Konasana

Supta means supine, lying on back. In supine, your knees in a bent position. This relaxes your inner thigh and groin muscles, and releases tightness. All your abdominal organs are stimulated. It also relaxes your mind and the central nervous system, which can bring about meditative quietness.

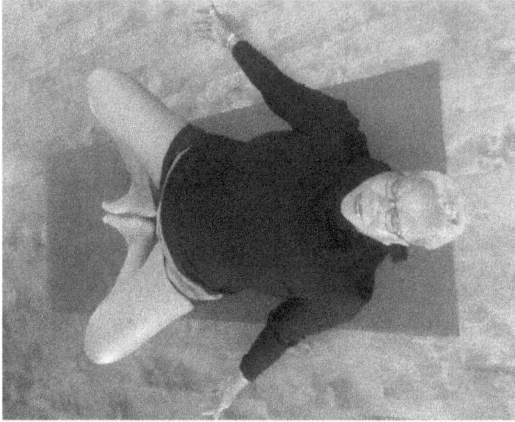

Lie flat, bend your knees, open your thighs, touch the soles of your feet together and place your palms up. Allow your knees to gently flow down towards the floor with each exhale. Each inhale can relax the thighs even more.

Meditating Sitting in Half Lotus

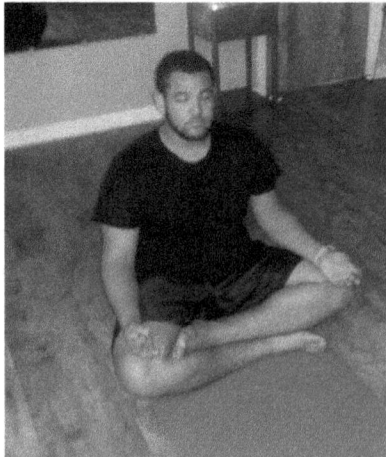

In Half-Lotus, with the thumbs and index fingers touching, the pranic energy (life force) is sealed from leaving the body.

The body forms a triangular shape where the energy circulates and stays within.

Actually, you can meditate anywhere, as long as you are not doing something dangerous like using heavy machinery or driving a car. Once you know how to quiet your mind, you can meditate while doing the dishes or vacuuming the floor, taking a hike or sitting in your favorite chair.

Devote at least twenty minutes (work up to an hour) sitting before your altar, seated on your bed, or in a chair. Practice any form of meditation or prayer that you are personally drawn to.

Sometimes what I do is light a candle or burn my favorite incense - Nag Champa or another soothing scent. You can put on music that soothes and inspires you, or use none. I don't always play music. Place meaningful objects, like flowers on your altar, and create a sacred circle around you with your intention. Call in your guides, angels, archangels, or your spiritual teacher.

Research from Dr. Joseph Mercola of the National Center for Complementary and Alternative Medicine (NCCAM) also supports the notion that: "Meditation acts as a form of 'mental exercise' that can help regulate your attention and emotions, while improving well-being. Even better, these changes may be permanent... It's been found previously that meditation prompts changes in the amygdala, a region of the brain associated with processing emotion. Newer research suggests these beneficial brain changes persist even after the meditation session is over, resulting in enduring changes in mental function."

Being still, you focus on your breath, joy, stillness and being present. Feel your breath, or feel the blood pumping through you, or focus on the candlelight. Release random thoughts; watch them leave you by your command. Detach from them.

Yogi Bharat taught me to focus on the breath. I've heard many times, that meditating is listening to God. "The mouth of God is the mind of man," as Neville Goddard has stated in his tapes and lectures. Prayer is speaking to God. So in meditating, you are breathing and listening and aligning to the Mind of God. You are listening to the silence and being in the silence and witnessing how it is and how it feels to be in that silence. Once you put a thought to it, that silence is gone.

By breathing in to the sound of OM (aum) and exhaling the same sound within your mind, you start to see that you are controlling your mind from wandering. You prevent it from getting involved with many thoughts or concerns trying to vie for your attention.

Make it your intention to eventually concentrate on a mantra like "Om Na-mah Shi-va-ya", "I Am that I Am", or just focus on the breath or the sound of OM as you sit quietly.

Half Lotus Beginner

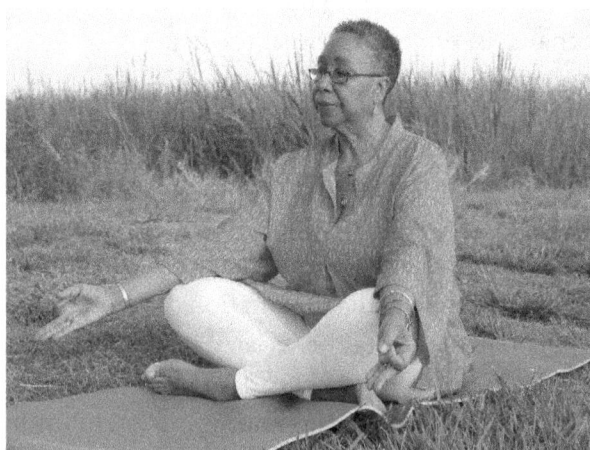

Place your thumb, representing truth and your index finger, which represents knowledge, against the thumb against the tip of the index finger. (Thumb and Index Fingers touch, others are extended into a yoga mudra (energy lock). This joining of the fingers means you are uniting with God. In the silence, you are one with God. Stretch the other fingers out straight, place your straight arms and hands to rest on your knees. This keeps your circuitry of energy flowing within and not dissipating away and out from you.

End your meditation by focusing the energy back into your body. Give thanks for this great blessing. Notice how you feel after your meditation and sense how light, but grounded you are.

If you are a smoker, anxious, can't sleep, worried or hyper, make it your intention to get your mind clear. Let yourself receive permission from within to meditate. You will get the answers you need to solve any problem, because you are the answer. God has revealed the answers for your inner self. You just need to sit and decide to listen; being patient and loving to yourself. Meditation is bliss. Give up trying to be God and BE God. Live God. Think God.

You will notice a change in the way you feel when finished. Your energy will be light and you will feel different about the way you see things. Thank your guides and release them on their way. I like to smooth my aura, swishing down and away, as I know I am bringing loving energy my way.

After meditation, if it is at night, you might drift off to sleep peacefully and release all cares, sending prayers to the Lord (Law) to be demonstrated the next day for you. If it's in the morning, practice your yoga asanas afterwards.

Personally, I don't put myself in a rut by doing the same thing every day. I listen to what I need to be doing by tuning in to my Inner Guidance.

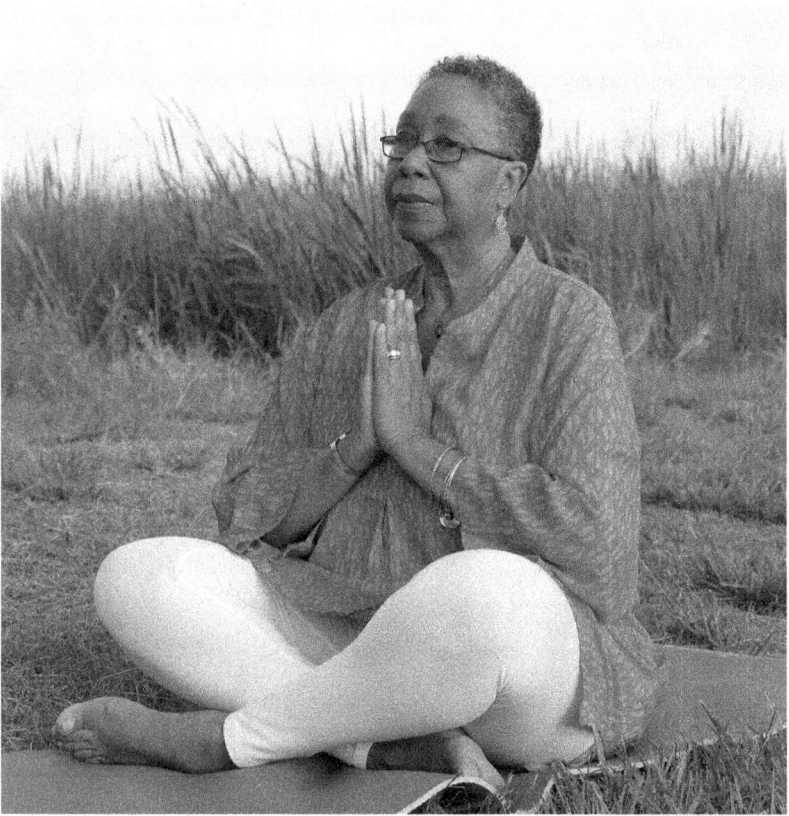

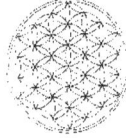

Chapter 6

Yoga and Health

*I AM Master of MYSELF. Remember always that the
"I" is the highest part of you that has been awakened into
consciousness, and should, to a great extent be master of the
animal nature from which you have emerged.*

~Yogi Ramachakara

Why Would Anyone Practice Yoga?

You might decide to practice because you heard from a friend of
yours that through her yoga practice she learned that it reduced
her stress and relaxed her body. She found it reduces the level of
the stress hormone cortisol through her research and she experienced the results. She told you that her digestive problems have
been erased or eliminated. Her conditions of anxiety, depression
or insomnia are no longer present. All these results have been
documented in yoga practitioners.

- **Pain Relief.** Many people have found pain relief is a by-product of the type of yoga they have been practicing. They may
  have found that by doing Power yoga; for example, it has
  been effective for them in erasing pain. Bikram Yoga has been
  beneficial for them because the heat you work under releases
  many toxins from the joints and body.

- **Increased Strength**, mentally and emotionally, is also a by-product of meditating. Being still and breathing slower brings about much clarity, peace of mind and higher self-esteem. With a yoga practice, it will help maintain weight management because you will burn calories gently.

- **Better Breathing.** Better breathing takes place when you learn to breathe properly. You take slower, deeper breaths. Relaxation is a natural result, which continues to blossom as you practice. The lungs improve their function, which increases the amount of oxygen (and pranic energy) to the rest of the body.

- **More Flexibility.** You become more flexible. The synovial fluid around the joints is increased for more cushioning of the joints. Muscles along the spinal column are lengthened, over time, with frequent practice. Muscles surrounding the joints and the bones are lengthened and become less tight, so bending is no longer a problem. Stomach muscles are firmer and tighter to act as a girdle for the abdominal cavity (the colon, large and small intestines). The organs and glands are gently stimulated.

- **Improved Circulation** is another reason to practice yoga. The yoga postures (asanas) effectively manage oxygen to flow more proficiently to the body's cells. All glands, organs, tissues, bones, blood, lymph fluids and spinal fluids are definitely affected and enhanced for the better. By yoga practice you can lower your resting heart rate over time and help issues with blood pressure as well.

- **Proper Body Alignment** is achieved through the use of postures. Aligning your body helps you to manage or eliminate back pain, joint and/or muscle problems, and neck or leg pain.

Having a yoga practice, one that you choose, which feels right for you, helps you to focus on the present and to live in the now. You tend to release worry about the future and remorse for the past. It helps you to be living happily in the present moment, which will create a bright future on its own.

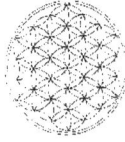

Chapter 7
Healing With Yoga

Life is for the fulfillment of our higher nature.
~ H. H. Swami Vishnu Devananda

Healing With Yoga

Yoga has been used for thousands of years because of its many and long lasting healthy benefits. Maintaining your youth, flexibility and healing can be done with yoga. The various styles of yoga, such as: Hatha Yoga, Iyengar Yoga, Ashtanga Yoga, Vinyasa Yoga, Kripalu Yoga, Bikram Yoga, Kundalini Yoga and other styles of Yoga, are extremely helpful and beneficial for body, mind and spirit.

The body systems, such as: the skeletal system, reproductive system, circulatory system, the endocrine glands, lymphatic system and organs are healed by the inversion asanas, stretching postures, back bend asanas and twisting asanas. These are great for the spine and vertebrae if there are back problems.

Taking time to relax in each posture, breathing properly and not forcing yourself beyond your limit, will make your Yoga practice enjoyable.

The therapeutic values of Yoga are realized by a routine yoga practice at home or at a yoga center or studio. Take the time to eliminate back pain gradually with a simple pose such as the Cat Cow Posture. There are at least 26 basic postures that can aid one who is dealing with back pain. You can find more at the Yoga Journal site or other Internet resources on this.

The cat-cow posture can increase strength to the muscles of your back and you will aid the spine in becoming more flexible, if done slowly with intention and purpose.

The cat-cow posture can increase strength to the muscles of your back and you will aid the spine in becoming more flexible, if done slowly with intention and purpose.

Cat Cow - Bidalasana

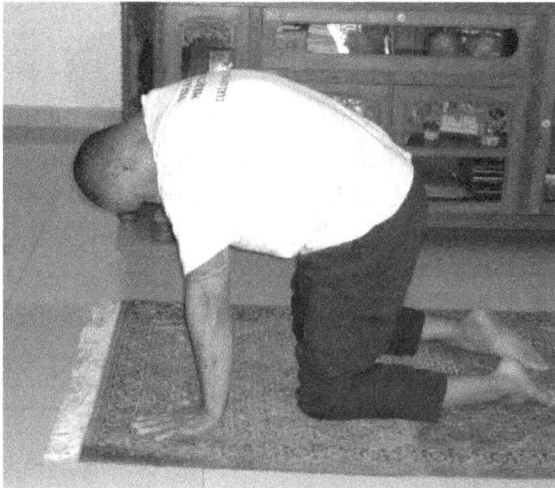

Inhale through your nostrils, hold your chin up, and push your tailbone out and away from your back. Place your knees in the table top position, rest your feet on the insteps, place your knees a hip-width apart.

Exhale as you pull in your abdomen to the spine, round your back and draw your chin down to your chest, with your arms straight, placing your palms flat onto mat. Repeat at least 5-10 times.

Learn how you can heal your body with yoga. Learn how you can maintain your health with yoga. There are two books, one being, *Ancient Secrets of the Fountain of Youth* by Peter Kelder and the other, *Your Hands Can Heal You* by Stephen Co and Eric B. Robbins, M.D. They are excellent books demonstrating how to regain youthfulness, flexibility and strength.

Yoga, as I have mentioned before, is about union, uniting the body, mind and spirit. Many times, the body responds to just being still and quiet, and the muscles will relax. Choose a form of yoga that feels right that you can relate to.

Healing with yoga can take 10 minutes a day, 30 minutes a day or longer. It's your choice. If you are a stay at home mother, you can invest in taking your style of yoga online. There are many excellent yoga instructors and you don't have to pack up diaper bags, formula, etc.

If you have limited mobility and you decide to attend the yoga school of your choice, let the teacher know before the class so he or she can modify the postures for you. Also be sure to check with your physician, if you have one, before attending a class.

Authors Peter Kelder, Stephen Co and Eric Robbins remind us that it's very necessary to keep the muscles and bones flexible and firm so that your blood can flow easily and effortlessly to all parts of the body. The lymphatic system and glands are stimulated by the soft motion of the postures.

By doing inverted postures (asanas), keeping the core or abdominal muscles firm and taut, keeping the upper legs firm and stretched and causing the spine to stay or become flexible, you become stronger and more mobile, and you feel more alive and healthy.

It is suggested by many yoga instructors to "Leave any frustration you might have at the front entrance of the yoga center or studio, and that will leave space for you to invite joy in its place." You should also apply this principle to your practice at home.

Mountain Pose Samasthiti or Tadasana

There are many benefits associated with the Warrior Poses, including: Strengthening your shoulders, arms, thighs, ankles and the muscles of your back; Expanding your chest, lungs and shoulders, Stretching your hip flexors, abdomen, and ankles; Developing stamina and endurance in your thighs and core muscles; Stimulating abdominal organs and digestion; and Improving your balance, concentration, and core awareness.

Warrior I - Virabhadrasana I

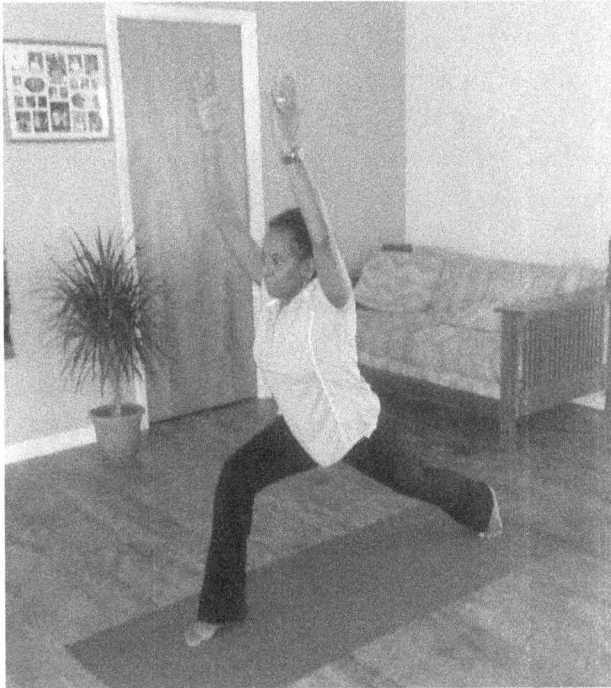

- Take a wide-legged stance, with your right foot straight ahead, and your right knee bent at a 90- degree angle.
- Hold your left foot parallel to your mat. Hold your arms up and raised, close to ears, and straight. Torso faces forward. Sink your torso down with a nice stretch. Don't forget to breathe nice and slowly.

- Take a wide-legged stance, with your left foot straight ahead, your left knee is bent at 90 degree angle. Your Right foot is parallel to your mat, with straight leg.

- Hold your arms up in airplane fashion, level with shoulders, body and hand face in the direction of your bent knee. To balance yourself, lean into your knee, and gaze at the middle finger of left hand. Don't forget to breathe nice and slowly. Be strong, feel your strength and power.

Warrior 2 - Virabhadrasana 2

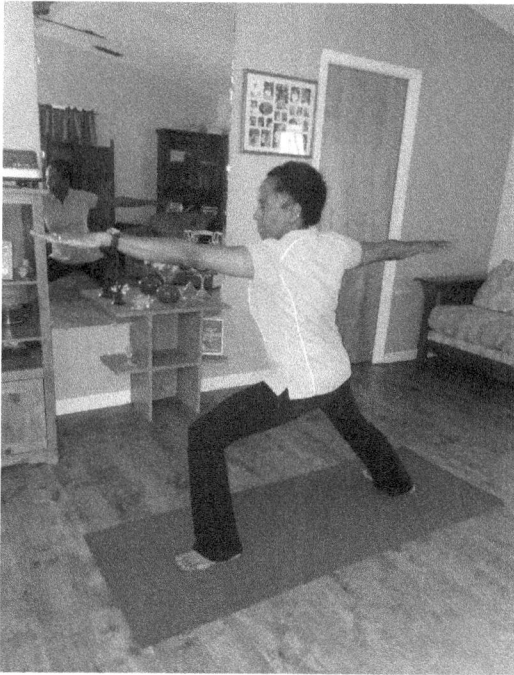

This pose strengthens the legs, thighs, hamstrings, tightens the core, arms, and balances while deepening concentration.

- Take a 3-4 foot stance, bend your right knee at a 90- degree angle, and push forward into the right thigh keeping your right knee just above your ankle in an "L" shape. Your back foot is parallel to your mat.

- Turn your torso sideways, raise your arms to shoulder level and face in the direction of your right knee. Gaze at the middle finger of the right hand as it is outstretched. Lean into your posture and feel free and strong with your breath.

Warrior 3 - Virabhadrasana 3

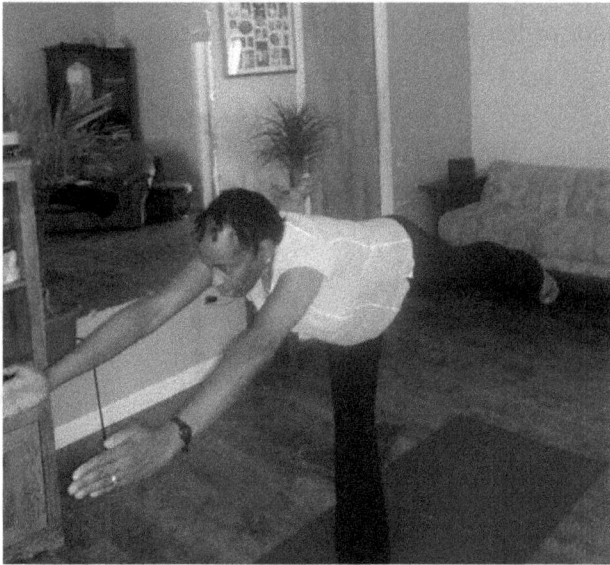

This pose balances and strengthens your arms and legs.

- You can move from Uttanasana (Standing Forward Bend), with your arms out in front, raise right or left leg back behind you as you grip your mat with your toes, grounding yourself to the floor.

- Gently focus on a spot in front of you to keep your gaze soft while you breathe. Lifting that back leg, keep focusing on breathing and balancing.

There are several variations of the Seated Forward Bend. Either one can be a challenging and strengthening pose for the hips.

It opens the hips, stretches the entire back side of the body, the legs and arms, and stretches the inside muscles of the legs. It also stimulates the abdominal organs, releases the groin muscles and strengthens the spine

Wide Legged Angle Seated Forward Bend (Upavistha Konasana)

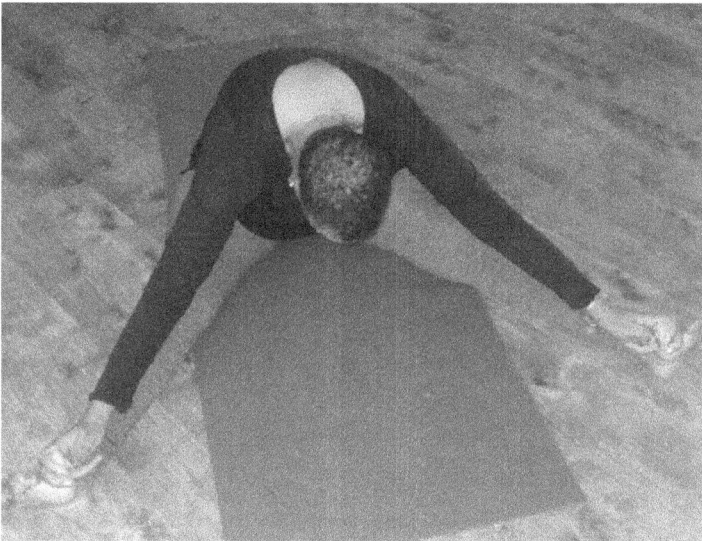

- Sitting in Dandasana, spread your legs wide apart as far as you can.
- Exhale and lean forward to touch your big toe, ankles, shins or knees, whichever you can reach. Breathe in quietly using ujjayi breath.

Seated Forward Bend - Paschimottanasana

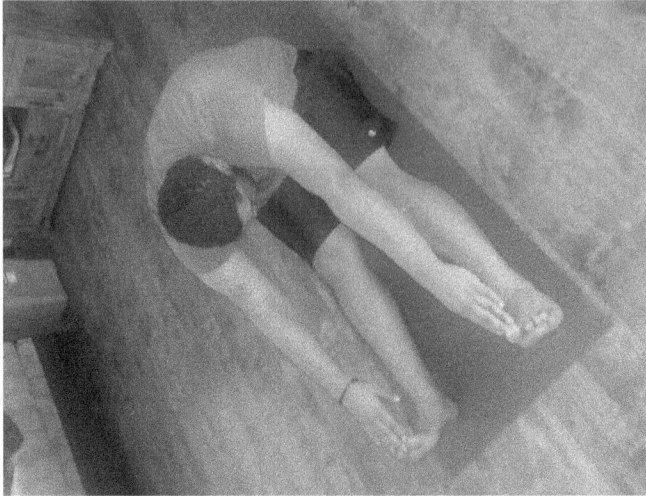

- Sitting in Dandasana, keep your legs together.
- Inhale deeply, lengthen your torso, exhale and fold forward to touch your shins, ankles, toes or whichever you can reach. Breathe in quietly using ujjayi breath. Work up to five inhalations.

Head to Knee Pose - Janu Sirsasana

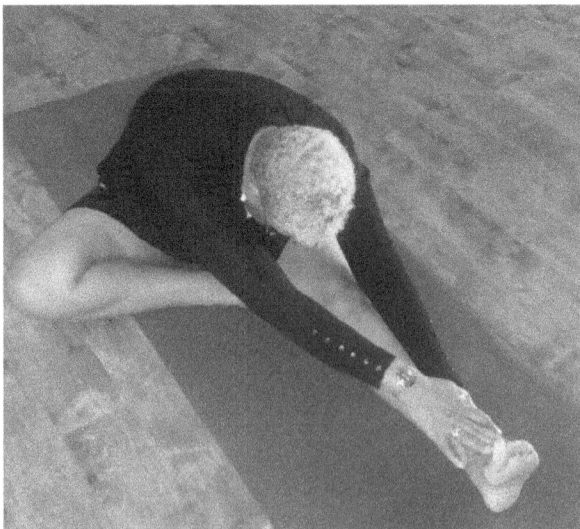

We start in Dandasana – Seated Staff Pose

- Sitting up straight, legs extended forward, bring your right or left leg up so the sole of your foot touches the inner thigh or groin area.
- Inhale, exhale and lean forward, stretch your arms together to touch the toes of your extended leg.
- Breathe in and out five times or five breaths. Feel what happens to your digestive system, the hamstrings and how your knees become more flexible with the synovial fluid in your knees being allowed to flow more easily now.

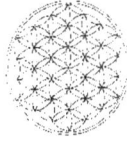

Chapter 8

Basic Points of Yoga Etiquette in a Class

Fate or destiny is your own creation through your own karmas. You are the master of your destiny. Change your mode of thinking from "I am the body" to "I am Atman, the all-pervading.

~Swami Sivananda

Basic Points of Yoga Etiquette in a Class

Here's how to make the class more enjoyable for all concerned, regardless of whether you are in a gym, studio or center.

- Respect the yoga space. Most all yoga centers, studios, and gyms have a place for your belongings, like your shoes, socks, bags, and other small items.
- Follow directions. There may be a special order for placing your mat on the floor.
- Come to class early enough so as not to disturb anyone else or the teacher. Keep chatting to a minimum once class starts. Inform your instructor if you have any health concerns or injuries.

- Don't push past your limits, maintain a good attitude, keep an open mind and breathe. Be courteous by remembering to turn off your cellphone before class begins.

- Be kind and avoid wearing heavy fragrances such as perfumes or aftershaves to a yoga class. Some people are allergic and not everyone enjoys "your" fragrance like you do; and it can be distracting and uncomfortable.

- Leave gum chewing at the door. Some people, like Oprah and I, are annoyed by smacking and cracking of chewing gum.

- If you have not pre-registered, please make class payment before class begins.

- If you eat before class, eat lightly, no less than one hour before class.

- Have clean bare feet, wear comfortable, yet loose-fitted clothes and bring a water bottle. You can bring your own personal mat, but most studios or centers have mats and props available for class.

- Please use good hygiene and no strong deodorants.

Sequence Suggestions for Hatha Yoga Beginners

Students should begin a sequence with simple poses. While each style of yoga has its own ideas about how to begin an asana practice, we all recommend to start with warm ups, and we value meditation and breathing techniques.

The basic sequence I use for students in Hatha Yoga is to begin with Savasana, the Corpse pose, for 5-10 minutes. I allow them to breathe and get centered when they come into class and rid themselves of outside thoughts, worries or concerns.

Corpse Pose - Savasana

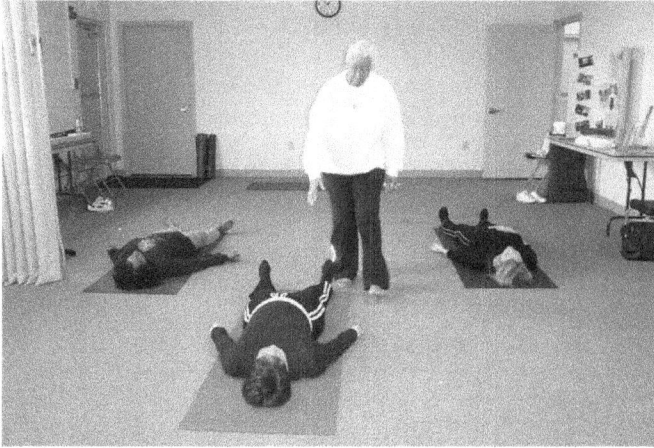

To get into the Savasana Pose, you should lay on the floor on your back with feet spread about twelve-inches apart, and heels on the corners of the mat. Place your arms and palms by your torso on each side. Center yourself on the floor with conscious breathing and exhaling through the nostrils.

You should then go to warm up poses (asanas) like hip openers, leg openers and leg warm ups. You may then want to into pranayama, mantras and chanting because the energy will deem it so, according to Spirit.

Then move to floor postures on the back, to stomach postures like the Locust, Bow, Cobra (Bhujangasana) or Upward Facing Dog, Plank and Side plank, while remembering to breathe the cleansing breath through each pose.

Then move into standing poses, such as the Eagle Pose (Garudasana), Triangle (Trikonasana) and variations of that, focusing on the spine at one point; hips and legs in another repetition; and then the Chair Pose (Utkatasana).

Eagle Pose - Garudasana

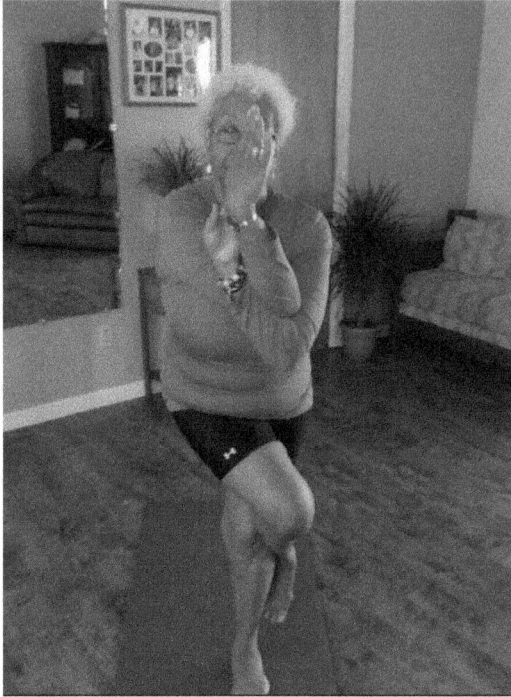

- Stand in your Tadasana Pose. Feet together. Relax and get centered.
- Cross your right arm over the left, bend the elbows. Touch the palms together flat, shoulders are opened and down away from your ears.
- Get your left foot grounded into your mat as if you had roots growing from the sole. Take your right leg, cross it close and over the left knee, wrap the right foot back behind the left leg as you gaze softly at a spot in front of you. Have your gaze about 2-inches away from your fingers.

Chair Pose - Utkatasana

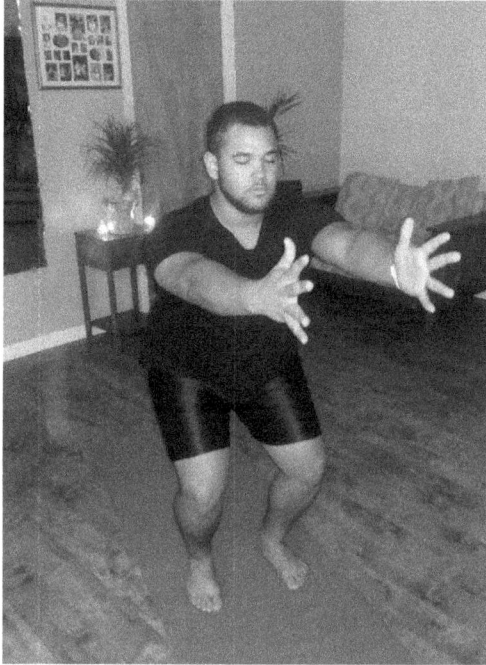

- Bring your arms out of Eagle Pose.
- Bend your knees to one half squat, feet are flat and hips are a width apart as you push your tailbone back and out behind you.
- Raise your arms overhead by your ears or parallel to your shoulders
- Uttanasana (forward bend), with hands on floor, look ½way up and fold 3 times with your breath.
- Bend knees, lift shoulders and come back to Tadasana (standing) or Utkatasana.

We might work into Sun Salutation known as Surya Namaskar with 2-3 repetitions and more for advanced students. Next could be seated postures or balancing poses while seated, such as the boat or front plank. More descriptions on getting into these poses will be given shortly.

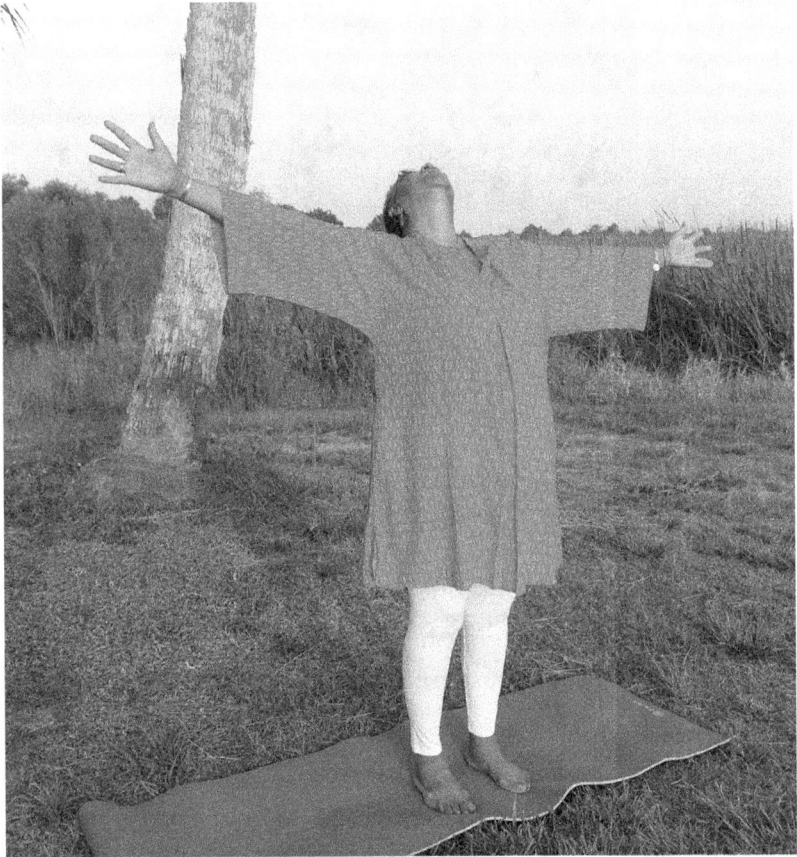

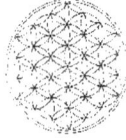

Chapter 9

Yoga & Weight Loss

I absorb from the Universal Supply of Energy, a sufficient supply of prana to invigorate my body – to endow it with health, strength, activity, energy and vitality.

~Yogi Ra Savasana macharaka

Yoga & Weight Loss

Can Yoga help with weight-loss? Yes. Yoga helps mental clarity, emotional clearing and cleansing; yoga helps to establish flexible muscles, joints and bones; and yoga helps with breathing, improved lung capacity, circulation and it can help with weight loss. If you do asanas once a week for only 5 minutes you will have little chance of making improvements. However, it doesn't take a huge amount of time. It's better if you take up Yoga ten to thirty minutes a day, every day or every other day…don't you think?

Once you decide to begin, there are asanas (postures) that you can utilize in your practice for firming up your buttocks and gaining strong legs. But if you don't use the techniques, how can you get results that you are imagining for yourself?

There are many five-minute glute and leg strengthening series, just as there are many five-minute weight loss postures that you can establish for yourself, at your own time and in your own special place.

I'll share some of the postures that can be utilized specifically for weight-loss, but just remember Yoga is not a one-sided process. One part of you doesn't get "cooked" and the other stays "undone". You need to take a balanced approach. You can choose to focus more on several postures, but do not exclude others.

Get into what's called Vinyasa or a Yogic flow using some of these postures such as, Boat pose, Navasana, Twisting poses, Warrior pose, Cat-Cow, Half Bridge, Cobra, Upward Facing Dog, Locust, Triangle and Reversed plank.

Half Bridge - Setu Bandhasana

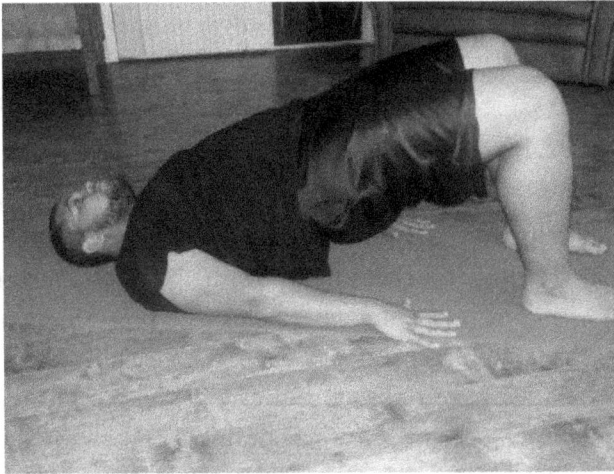

- Lie on your back, with arms alongside torso, palms pressing down on mat. Shoulders open, take deep inhale, and lift your buttocks from the mat. Keep your knees a hips-width apart and feet flat on the mat. Breathe in at least 5 times.

The following postures are fat-burning and energizing and are pretty simple to accomplish at home. Do a repetition of five times with five inhalations and five exhalations for each repetition. Remember to breathe utilizing the Ujjayi breath (through nostrils) that is taught under the Pranayama section.

You'll see the next students preparing to move into some very common and helpful asana for the spine and abdomen. The student will inhale, pushing back the tailbone and lifting it up a bit, while raising the chin up slightly.

6. The shoulders will be open wide with palms directly under the shoulders. After exhaling, round your back by pulling in the tummy and tucking the tailbone under. Do 5-10 repetitions.

Preparing for Cat Cow Posture - Bidalasana

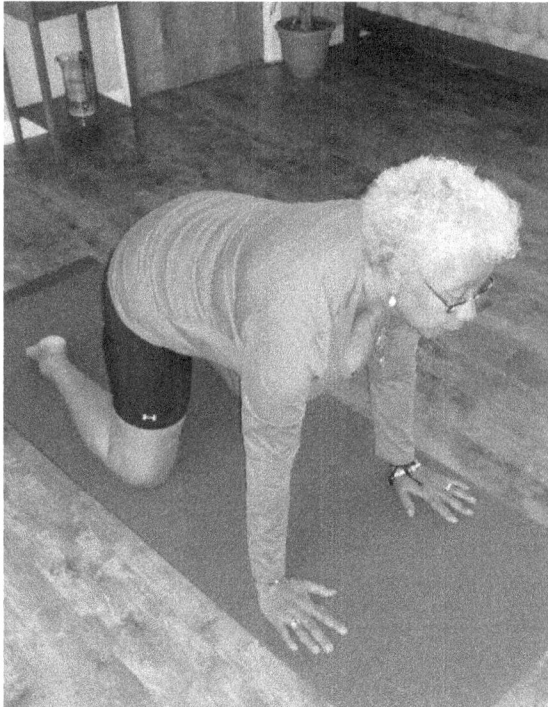

After you do the Cat-Cow known as Bidalasana, you can gently move into Upward Facing Dog posture (Svanasana).

Upward Facing Dog - Urdhva Mukha Svanasana

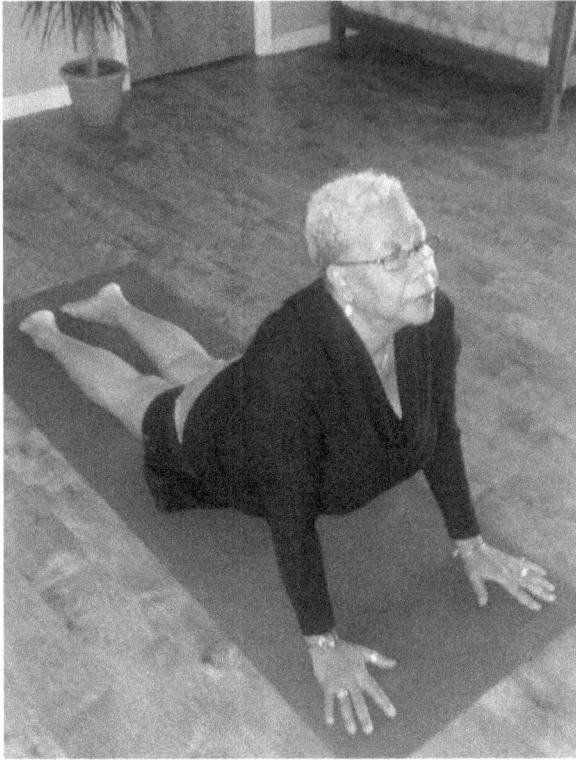

Lengthen out your legs behind you, with insteps on the mat or toes curled under, whichever is more comfortable. If the arms are strong enough, you can lift your thighs off the mat while breathing in and out through your nostrils, holding your head up. Otherwise you can rest on your knees or knees and thighs. Arch your back very slightly helping to strengthen your spine, abdomen and buttocks. Keep your shoulders open.

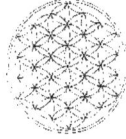

Chapter 10

Yoga Basics & Tips for a Great Yoga Practice

"I used to lose all the time, but after learning this technique of meditation, I now win almost all the time. I meditate, I detach, and I don't worry about the result and jump into my competition."

~ Olympic Winner

Yoga Basics

Seated poses, standing poses, twist poses, supine poses, inverted poses and balance poses all help increase circulation, stimulate the brain, enhance glandular system functioning and relieve pressure on the abdominal organs.

They help relieve you of stress, toxins and negative mental energy through movement, meditation and your intention. Yoga and breathing, breath awareness exercise, abdominal breath, three-part breath are all necessary in your Yoga practice; to firm, tone, heal, stay alert and energize. There are many resources available regarding Yogic breath.

There are several poses that you can do to get all your muscles stretched and the blood flowing nicely.

Warm-up Poses

- Neck rolls and stretches
- Shoulder Stretches
- Arm Stretches
- Spinal Roll
- Rock the Baby
- Leg raises
- Little Boat Pose
- Pigeon Pose
- Squat Pose

Standing Balancing Poses:

- Dancer Pose Natarajasana
- Tree Pose
- Standing Hand to Toe Pose
- Eagle Pose
- Half Moon Pose
- Triangle pose (Trikonasana)
- Chair posture (Utkatasana)

Dancer's Pose - Natarajasana

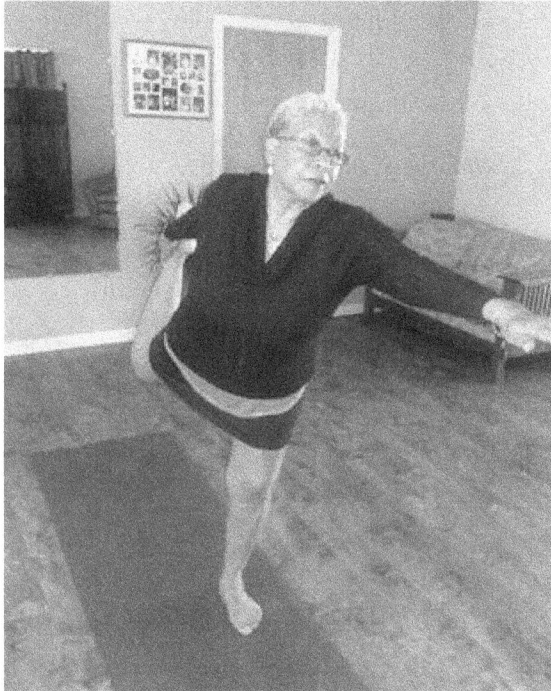

This is not a beginner's pose but can give you an idea of what to look forward to for yourself, with practice.

- The left foot grips the mat gently as you stand in Tadasana.
- Raise your left arm level to your shoulder or higher while you arch your back.
- Bring your right knee up towards your chest and bend your right leg behind you taking your right hand and grasping the outside or inside of your ankle, whichever is easier.
- Push your right leg back away from your body keeping your balance.
- Focus softly on something in front of you and breathe.
- Have your left palm facing the floor or take on what's called a yoga mudra (a hand finger position). Try to hold the pose for five breaths – or work up to it with two to three inhalations.

These are balancing, strengthening and grounding poses:

- Standing Forward Bend
- Right Angle Pose
- Standing Wide Angle Forward Bend

Standing Wide Angle Forward Bend - Prasarita Padottanasana

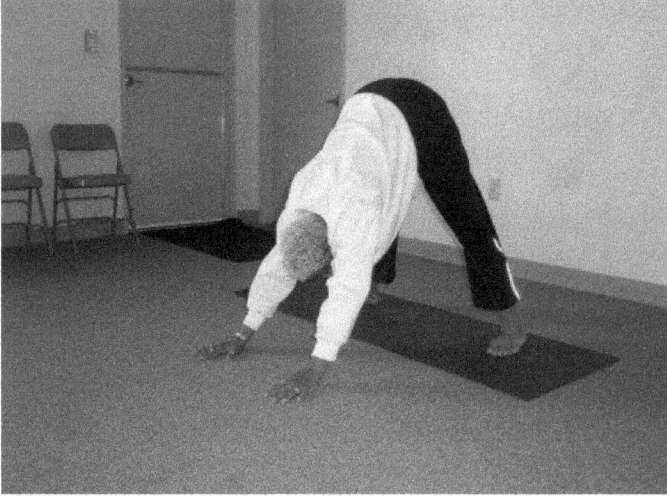

- Modified, wide-legged standing forward bend. Spread legs apart about three feet. Your feet are facing forward.
- Exhale as you bend from the waist, palms facing down. Your tailbone is pushed back and away up and out from body after the forward bend.
- Your back is flat and palms are flat pushing down onto the floor. Your head is between your straight arms. Breathe in through nostrils, using the Ujjayi breathing about five times as you relax the hips at the same time.

These postures get the vertebrae in alignment:
- Standing Forward Bend Twist
- Side Angle Twist
- Pyramid Pose
- Seated Spinal Twist
- Triangle Twist
- Rag Doll Pose

Seated Spinal Twist - Ardha Matsyendrasana

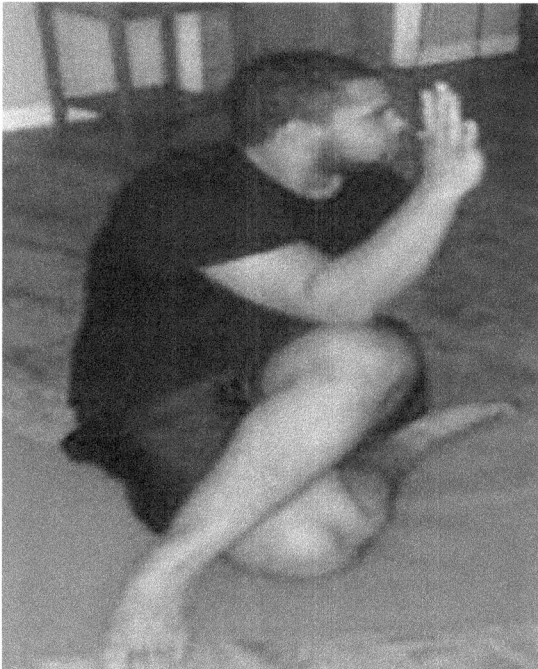

This asana works on spinal flexibility and stretching the muscles of the hips and lower back. This posture gets the vertebrae in alignment, strengthens the muscles surrounding them and the spinal column.

- Sitting on your mat, bend your right leg and bring your foot as close to your buttocks as you can.

- Cross your left leg over the knee on the floor, with your foot flat on the mat.

- Place your left hand behind you on the floor or use your fingertips.
- Twist spine with inhale towards the right. Place left elbow on the right knee, hand straight up with fingers pointing up towards ceiling with firmness. Turn head in direction of right shoulder slowly turning. Do both sides of the body.
- Twist your body as you are exhaling to the left, chin and head are level. Grab your left knee with your right hand pulling left knee towards you.
- Each exhale, you should be able to twist to the left more each time. Come out gently and repeat on the opposite side.

Kneeling Asanas
- Table Pose
- Cat Stretch
- Lunge Pose
- Thread the Needle Pose
- Plank Pose
- Downward-Facing Dog Pose

Table Pose - Four Limb Pose

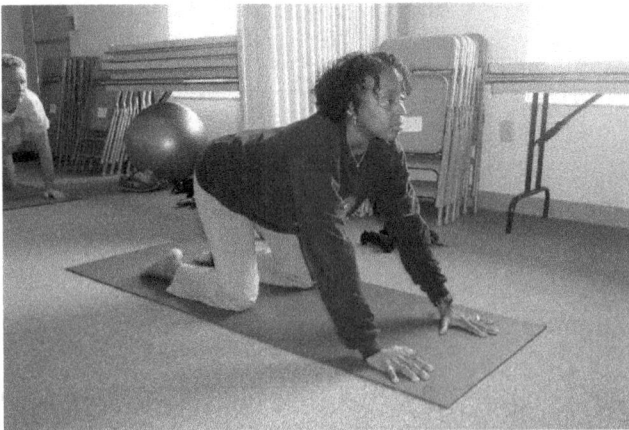

- Come to a kneeling position on hands and knees, palms firmly planted flat on the floor, shoulders over the wrists.

- Hips, should be a shoulder-width apart, arms the same. Arms are below the shoulders. Your back is flat and your head should be level with your spine. Do not hold your breath, use the pranayama of Ujjayi .

You are now ready to move from table position into cat-cow asana. As you inhale using the Ujjayi breath.

Cat Cow Pose - Bidalasana

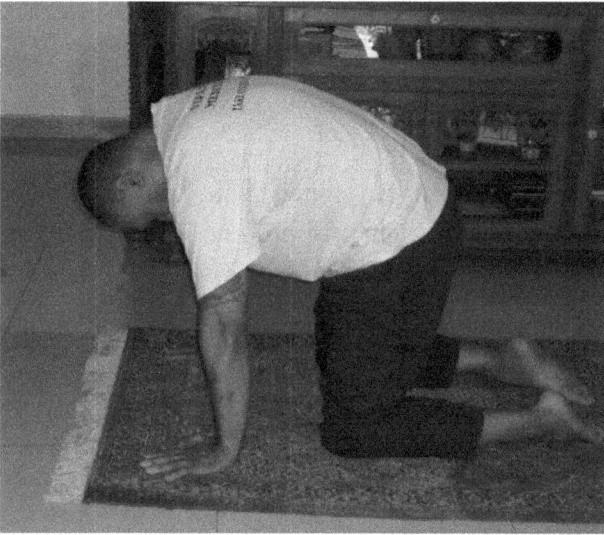

- Push the tailbone out and back away from you, sway the spine into a dip, chest up and open and chin moves up slightly.

- Exhale as you round the spine and round the tailbone tucking it in and lower the head, chin lowered as far as you can towards your sternum.

- Repeat this repetition 5-7 times.

Front Plank Pose - Reversed Purvottanasana

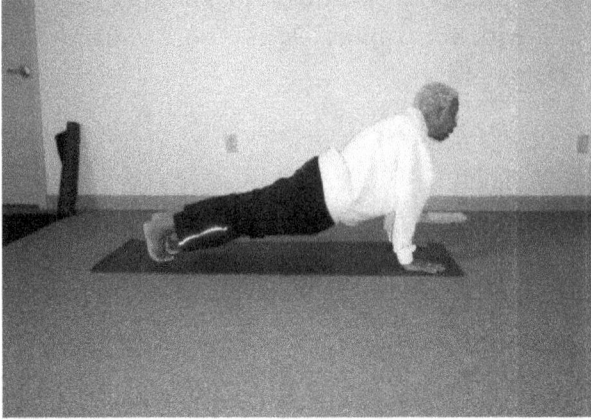

From cat-cow asana, you can stretch the legs back behind you, curls the toes under, legs straight and head is lined up with spine and heels. Arms directly under shoulders, lined up with wrists moves you into Front Plank Pose below.

Feel how beautiful this opening feels to you. No need to rush. This develops strength in your arms, tightens your core, legs and keeps you balanced and aware.

Upward / Reversed Plank - Purvottanasana

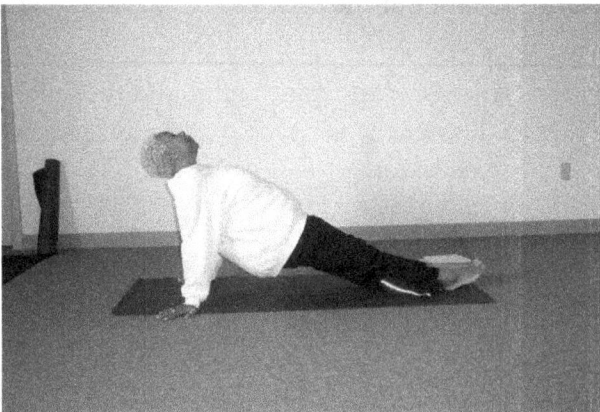

- Your head, spine, buttocks and heels should be in straight line, buttocks not sticking upward but level with head. Be one with your posture, breathe nice and slowly and keep your energy flowing.

- Move into Upward//Reversed) Plank or inclined position, head in alignment with back, legs and feet.

The following asanas are just a sample of what you can eventually put into your practice regardless of your age and initial flexibility. To begin seated postures, you can sit in Dandasana, seated staff pose, legs straight ahead on floor.

Seated Pose - Dandasana

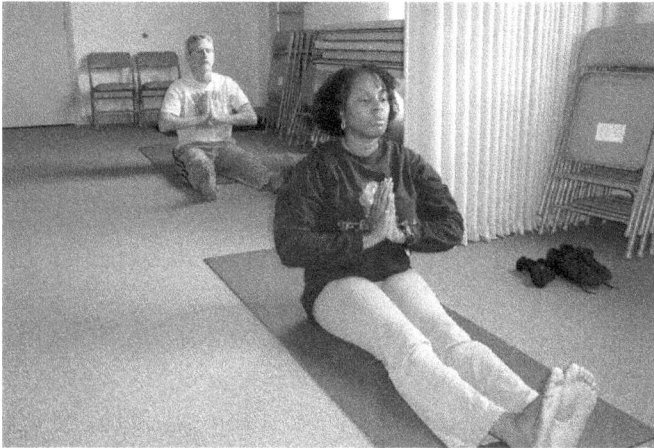

- Place your hands in Namaste position where they are at center of heart, palms touching.
- Feel the rhythm of your breathing and heartbeat. Center yourself.
- Straight back, hands to center of heart or placed behind or along each hip

Seated Staff Pose – Dandasana

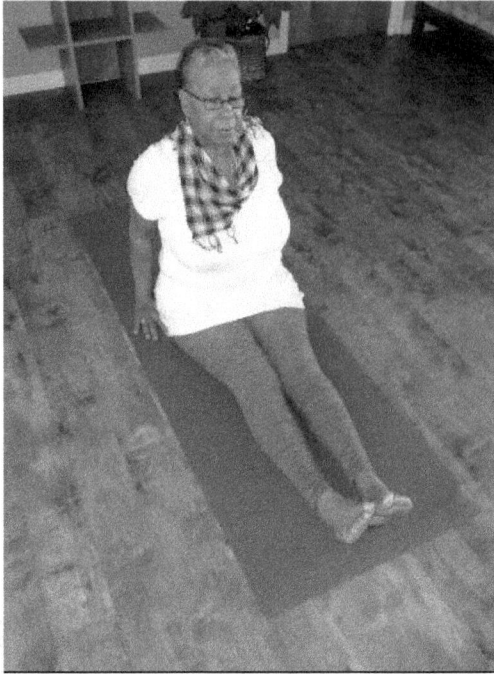

Start in Dandasana – Seated pose, legs are extended. Be one with your posture, breathe slowly and keep your energy flowing. Make sure your hips are lifted up. Breathe and relax for as long as you feel comfortable.

- After you place your hands on each side on the body on your mat and directly under shoulders behind you with your palms flat, as you lift the hips off the floor, legs extended, toes pointing together.
- Lift your chin as you breathe. Relax and breathe and gently come down on exhale after about three-five inhalations.
- Sitting up straight, with your legs extended forward, bring right or left leg up so sole of the foot touches the inner thigh or groin area.
- Inhale, exhale and lean forward, stretch your arms together to touch toes of extended leg.

- Breathe in and out five times or five breaths. Feel what happens to your digestive system, the hamstrings and how your knees become more flexible with the synovial fluid in your knees being allowed to flow more easily now.

- Your right knee is bent so the sole of the foot touches the inner left thigh.

- Breathing in, you exhale through the nostrils and take the outstretched arms and hands and lower your hands to ankles, instep or touch the sole of your left foot.

- Make it your intention to touch your knee with your forehead, keeping the back flat as much as you can.

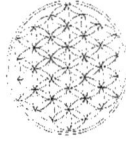

Chapter 11
Poses that Heal Joints

I have crossed from the wilderness of this world, into the Promised Land of plenty.

~Chris Doolin

Poses that Heal Joints

Start in Dandasana, close your eyes and sit with straight back, legs extended and feet together. Hands at heart center in Namaste position. After several centering breaths, move into the Table Pose.

Come from the Table Pose into Threading the Needle Pose shown below.

Threading the Needle Pose

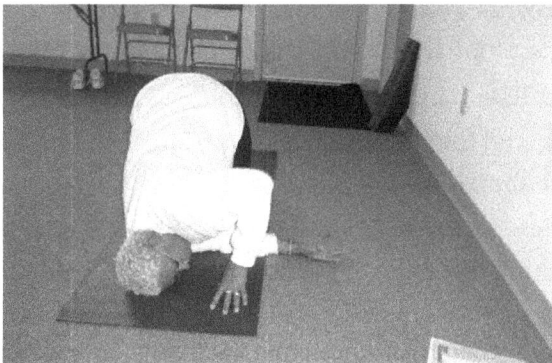

- Move from the Table Pose by taking your right arm and sliding it under the left arm that is up at right angle. Touch fingertips of left hand onto the mat. Right shoulder is now on the mat, right side of head is on floor.
- Push tailbone out behind you. Left elbow is up and breathing is easy through the nostrils about five inhalations. Switch sides. Be one with the breath.

Cow Posture – Gomukasana

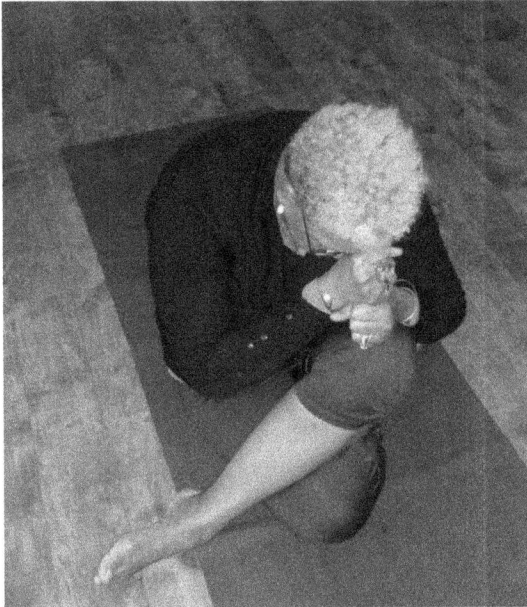

For Cow Posture, (Gomukasana), bend your knees and crisscross your legs, left foot close to the right thigh and the right foot close to the left thigh.

- Inhale and fold forward from torso after exhaling and pulling the abdomen in.
- Reach your forehead to the top of knees. Breathe and relax, breathing through your nostrils the ujjayi breath, mentioned under pranayama. You can stack your fists one on top of the other on the upper knee and touch your forehead to the fist.

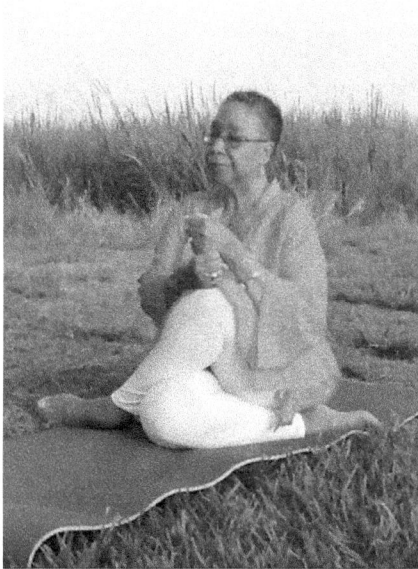

- Variation is extending your right arm up, bending it at elbow and reaching down behind your spine. The left hand goes back behind your back, reaching up to touch or grab the fingers of your right hand that is pointing downward along spine.

Back Bends

- Standing Back Bend
- Sphinx Pose
- Cobra Pose (Bhujangasana)
- Upward Facing Dog Pose
- Front Lying Boat Pose
- Half Locust
- Locust Pose
- Bow Pose
- Bridge Pose
- Fish Pose

Cobra - Bhujangasana

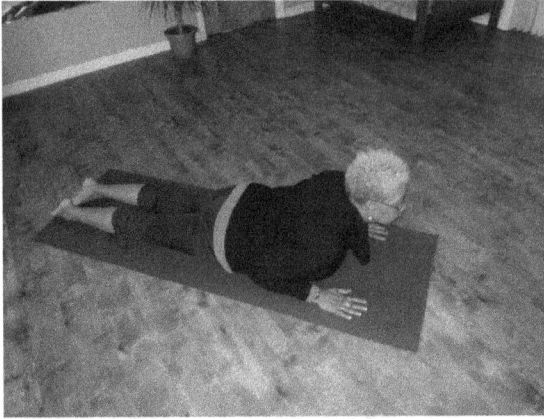

For the Cobra, lay on your tummy. Legs are extended back behind you, insteps touch the mat. Forehead is on the floor, palms are under the shoulder joint, arms are close by the ribcage, tucked in.

- Breathe in and press down on your palms, pushing your chest up very slowly, matching the breath. Feel that each vertebra is getting in alignment as you inch up. Arch your back as you move.

- Exhale and come down slowly as each vertebra is affected.

Move into Upward Facing Dog (Urdhva Mukha Svanasana) from Cobra by pushing up onto your palms, and then extend your arms so they are under your shoulders. Push up and move into Upward Facing Dog with legs extended back and behind you with insteps touching the mat.

Or you can come down from the plank posture onto your knees if you are just learning this. Otherwise hands and wrists are directly below the shoulders. Thighs are held up from the floor, toes are curled under or the insteps can be touching the floor. Keep your shoulders wide and open, chest up and head up away from the shoulders. Press down firmly with your palms and breathe about five inhalations, or work up from 2 inhalations to five.

Locust Pose - Salabhasana

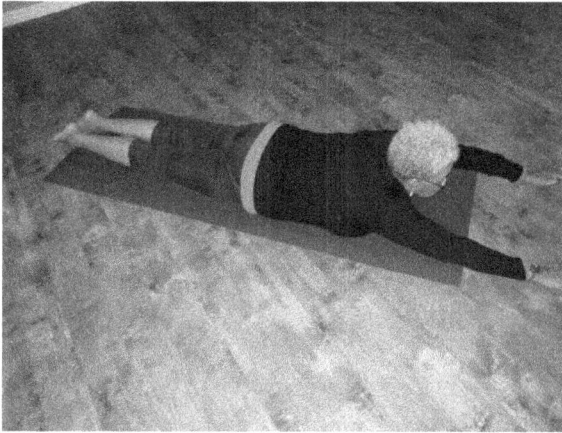

You can also easily move from the Cobra to a posture that strengthens the spine, thighs, legs and arms, which is called the Locust or Salabhasana.

- Just take the hands that were under your shoulders in Cobra and place them under your thighs, or you can stretch your arms forward.

- Then raise your head up at the same time you raise your lower legs, arching your back while you breathe and inhale. Your hands will help you to keep balance and encourage the leg raise to be a bit easier if they are placed palms up under your thighs.

- Breathe in deeply through nostrils, mouth is closed. Raise the arms and legs off the floor at the same time, chest open wide, shoulders back, or place arms on each side of the hips, palms touching side of thighs and chin is up.

- Exhale when ready and come back to the mat with your head resting on your hands in what is called the Crocodile Pose. There are additional Locust poses to suit your mobility, such as placing your palms under your thighs and using them to help lift up your thighs off the mat.

- Raise your head, shoulders and legs off the mat, together as you inhale.

Child Pose - Balasana

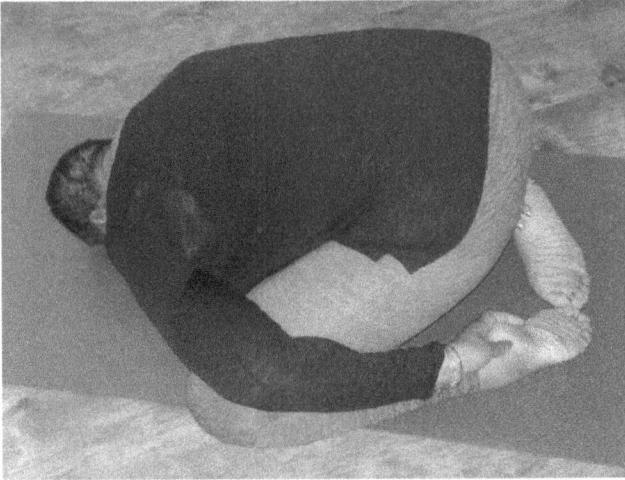

In the Child Pose, there can be at least a few variations of arm placement, based on what is comfortable for you and variation and flexibility where your hips are in relation to your heels. Move at your own flexibility and mobility.

- You can place your toes together, spread your knees apart into "v" shape and lower your buttocks onto your heels. In one version, you place your arms above your head onto your mat.

- In the other version, you place your arms and hands by your feet as you rest on your heels your forehead on the mat.

- From the Table Pose, you can move into the child asana by resting back onto your heels with your buttocks touching your heels. Spread your knees apart, with your toes touching. Lean forward to touch your forehead to the floor in front of you. *This is a very meditative pose and also a pose of gratitude.*

- Stretch your arms ahead of you resting them onto the floor or bring your arms back around the sides, with your hands touching your ankles, and your shoulders and spine relaxed.

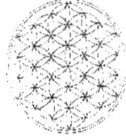

Chapter 12

Asanas are Suitable for Everyone

Asanas make one firm, free from maladies and light of limb.
~ Pradipika.

Asanas are Suitable for Everyone

There is no age limit for those who wish to practice yoga, or asanas, as the yoga postures are called. They can be practiced at any age, no matter whether you are 5 or 95.

Asanas are performed slowly with concentration, while taking deep, conscious breaths. The yoga postures strengthen the body and have positive effects on the body, mind and soul.

Beneficial for the Body, Mind and Soul

The yoga postures improve the flexibility of the spine and the joints, and strengthen the body's muscles, glands and internal organs. The body is invigorated and toned, and regains its ideal form.

Regular asana practice releases hitherto unknown sources of energy and leads to a whole new feeling of physical well-being.

The gentle movements also have a deep spiritual benefit: they help us to overcome fear, develop trust and find inner-peace.

Celebration

Allow yourself to be dictated to by your Higher Consciousness, your Higher Self known as the *I am Presence*. Allow yourself to receive the answers you are searching for.

Find your purpose, your passion. Allow yourself to make your passion work for you and through you. Give of yourself lovingly and freely.

Love yourself and find 100,001 ways to celebrate your being-ness here on earth. Find 100,001 ways or 10x that for being in the realm of gratitude!

Instead of believing in your personal lie any longer, believe now that, **"I am strong; I am a winner; I am through with being a victim."** Repeat those words aloud to yourself with feeling!!

At that precise moment, you have stepped over into the Realm of Freedom. All the answers you need to follow through with this new belief will come pouring in rapidly.

Thoughts that keep you away from seeing the face of God, out of the healing vibrational frequency of light, bliss, freedom and love are displaced with truth.

Finish these incomplete statements:

*I believe*_____

*I feel*_____

*I think*_____

*I doubt*_____

*I am afraid that*_____

*If only I could*_____

*Meditate on being*_____

Only in the Silence can you hear all things because

_____

Beginner and Intermediate Exercises

Some of the basic asanas as practiced in a classic yoga class are:

- Standing Forward Bend Twist
- Side Angle Twist
- Sphinx Pose
- Seated Spinal Twist
- Triangle Pose

Triangle Pose – Trikonasana

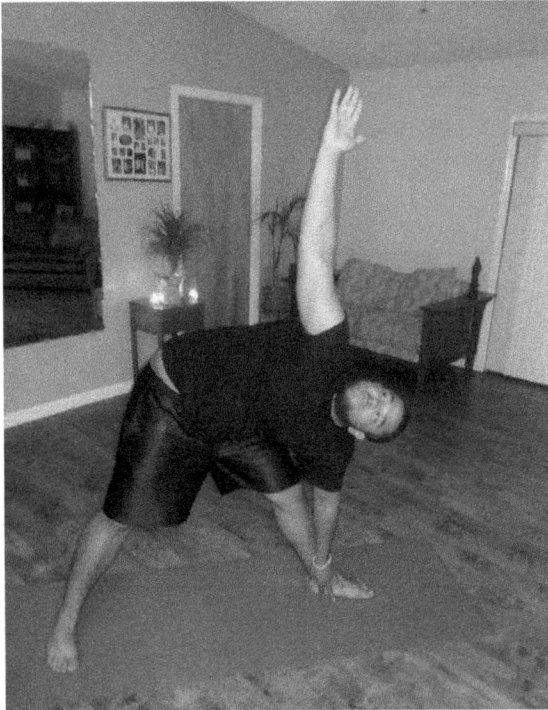

- Get into a strong, 3-4 foot wide stance
- Turn the left foot straight ahead of you while your back foot is parallel to the mat. Check to see if there is an invisible string linking the heel of the left foot to the middle of the back foot.
- Push out the right hip to the right side, then exhale and lower your left arm to your left ankle or foot.

- Your left hand can be placed behind your left foot or in front of your left foot.

- Stack the right shoulder over the left shoulder in as straight an invisible line as possible. Turn your head to face the right arm/hand. What else? Breathe and relax hips.

Kneeling asanas

- Table Pose
- Extended Cat Stretch
- Lunge Pose
- Eye of the Needle
- Plank Pose
- Downward-Facing Dog Pose

Eye of the Needle

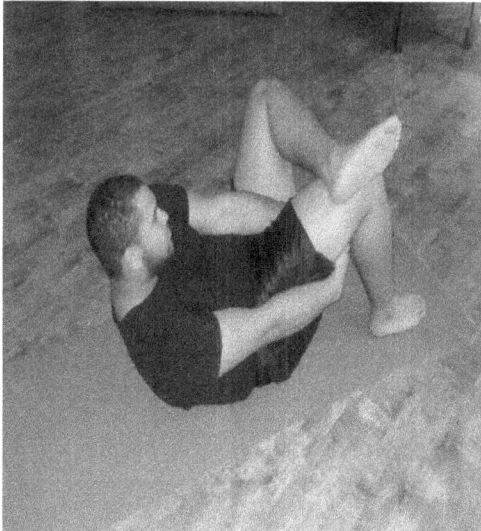

Eye of the Needle Pose is a relaxing way to soothe and remove stiffness from the hips and lower back muscles and joints.

- Lie on your back, cross your left leg over your thigh and rest the heel on the thigh or knee.

- The right knee is bent with your foot on the floor or raised off the floor.
- Thread your left arm through the space, wrap your right arm under the right thigh or around the right thigh, pull that knee close to your chest and clasp your fingers together.
- Raise your head with your inhale.

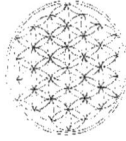

Chapter 13

A Sample at Home Asana Practice

Infinite Intelligence reveals to me ALL I need to know at all times!

~Daya Devi-Doolin

Illumination

Whether sitting, standing or kneeling, or before beginning any asana, become ONE with your breath.

1. With each inhale let your breath go in deeper and fuller and relax totally with each exhale.
2. Breathe – Ahhhhhh with each exhale.
3. Feel the Silence of your divine light.
4. Be light inside and outside.
5. Turn your awareness to the Silence within.
6. Let your body expand.
7. Feel the light of consciousness behind what you are doing.
8. Become filled with enthusiasm, joy, radiance and thankfulness.
9. Experience how freeing you feel, how happy you are.
10. Notice any freedom from darkness or negativities.

Warm ups

Just take two postures to begin with then work towards five.

Child's Pose- on your knees, with your buttocks tucked under and resting on your heels, with your arms outstretched, place your hands on the mat with your spine relaxed.

Do Crescent Lunge - bend your right knee at a 45-degree angle, place your back foot parallel to the mat, with your arms up towards the ceiling and close to your ears, arch your back and your fingers are spread out. Breathe in the light.

Come back to Down Dog and again to Crescent Lunge, Anjanyasana

Do Down Dog, then lightly jump to Uttanasana (forward bend) by bending your knees, come up on your tip toes, round your spine and hop towards your hands for the forward bend Uttanasana.

Down Dog - Ardha Mukha Svanasana

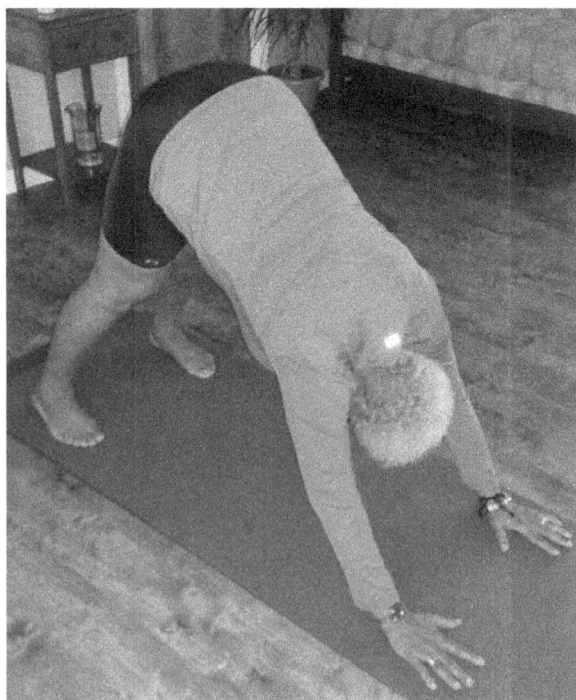

Slowly come up from Uttanasana, with your arms limp, rounded shoulders and back as you inhale and exhale until you are standing in Tadasana.

Sun Salutation or Surya Namaskar can be done instead of the above warm ups and repeated 2-3 times until you master it, standing facing the east.

How Can I possibly Learn the Sun Salutation (Surya Namaskar)?

You will learn the Sun Salutation by doing and practicing two poses at a time. When you feel it start to flow for you with those two, add one more and one more. We start above in the Namaste' hand position in Tadasana, sometimes called Samasttihi. Place your alms together, touching the heart center. There is an animated sequence on the Internet under ABC Yoga Sun Salutation referenced for you in my appendix of websites.

Sun Salutation (Surya Namaskar is comprised of 12 asanas and works the abdominal core metabolism, muscles, waist, and legs, circulatory, skeletal, respiratory, organs and glands. Bring your attention to your breath and become aware of your effortless breathing rhythm. Turn your mind off.

When you realize how important an effect these twelve poses can have on all your glands, organs, muscles and bones, heart and respiration, you will look forward to doing anything you can or how many postures you can until you increase the full number of poses.

Do not look at it as a daunting project. Look at it as loving yourself through motion and breath.

Generally, when you do Surya Namaskar you stand facing to the rising sun.

Mountain Pose - Tadasana

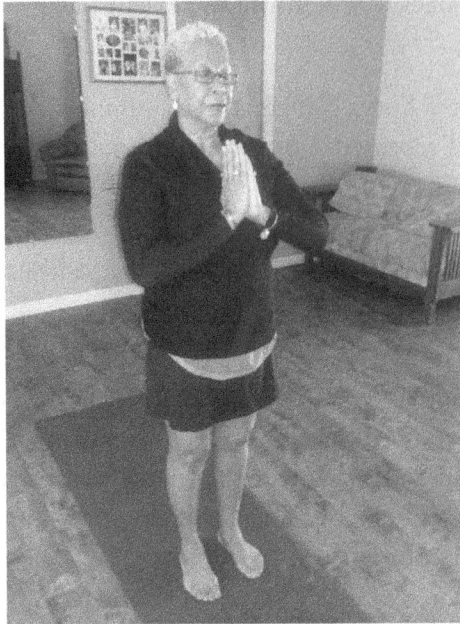

1) The first posture is to stand in what's known as the Mountain pose, Tadasana or Samasthiti, planting the feet solidly on your mat. Tilt your pelvic area forward a little, ever so slightly bend your knees.

Once you feel yourself centered and composed, bring your hands to your chest or heart center in prayer fashion or Namaste'. With your feet together, breathe and feel yourself become balanced, centered and free of anxieties. Breathe in a deep breath through the nostrils as you raise your arms overhead, touching your palms together. Open your arms apart with your in-breath, opening to grace and thankfulness and lean backwards by arching your back and pulling your head back as well.

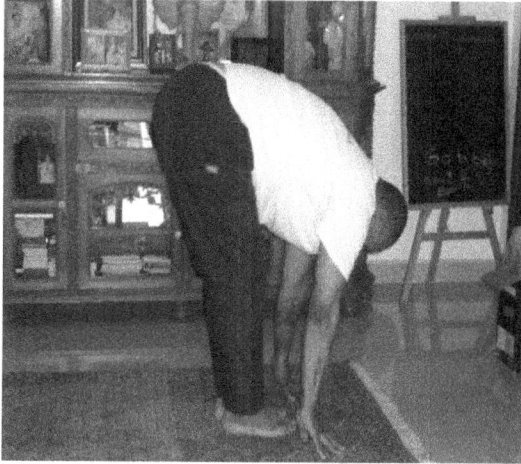

2) Next, exhale as you bend at the hips and lower your arms and hands to the tops of your feet.

Your hands can go around your ankles, or touching the shins, or even placing your hands beside or on top of your feet is fine. Whatever your level of flexibility is - listen and follow your body. Keep breathing in and out and bring your head closer and closer with each exhale to your knees. This really stretches and elongates the spine. You can give yourself permission to bend your knees slightly.

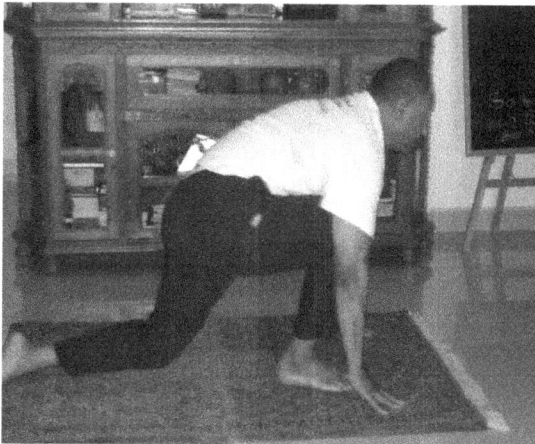

3) The next posture we'll move into of Surya Namaskar is placing the left leg back behind you while you bend the right leg at

a forty-five degree angle so it looks like an L-shape. That way no pressure is put on the knee.

The instep of your left foot can be touching the floor, or your foot can be placed on the floor at a 90-degree angle. Breathing in here is very important. There is no set amount of time in this pose.

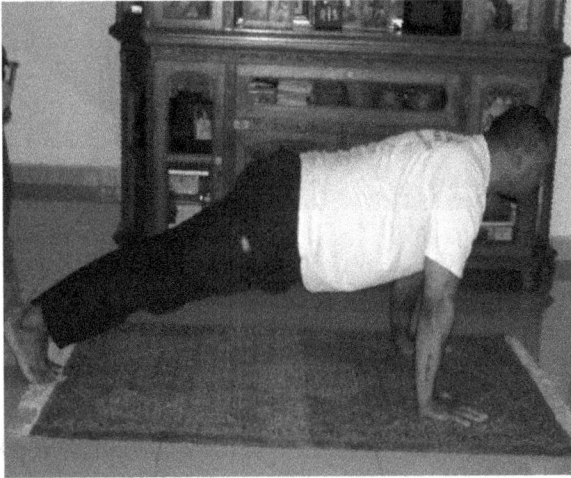

4) Now bring your right leg back to join the left leg and you will be in the Plank Asana.

Your chin is up and your hips are lowered, not sagging. Your body looks like a slant board. Your hands are flat on the mat with your shoulders opened.

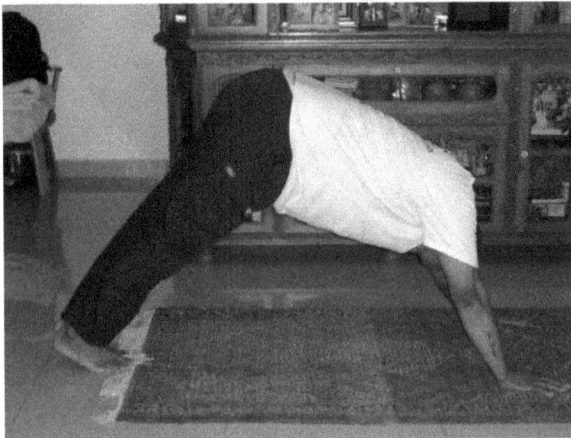

5) Your arms are directly under your shoulders. If this is your first time - just rest by lying down now or move into the Child's Pose.

From the plank pose, bend your knees together, place them on your mat, bring your chest to touch the floor at the same time, bending at the elbows, touch your hands to the floor beside you and your forehead.

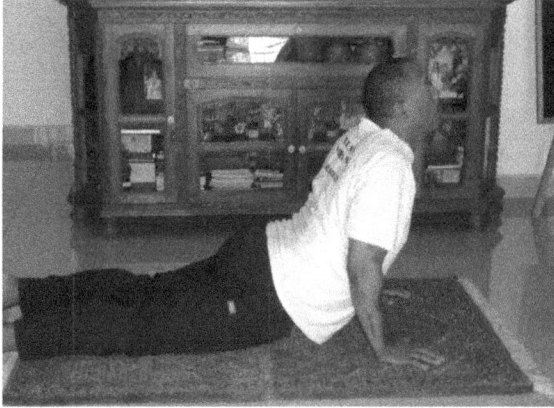

6) Move next to sliding gently into Upward Facing Dog, with your chest open wide down, away from your ears. Do the Upward Facing Dog with your thighs off the mat or on the floor, if not experienced enough.

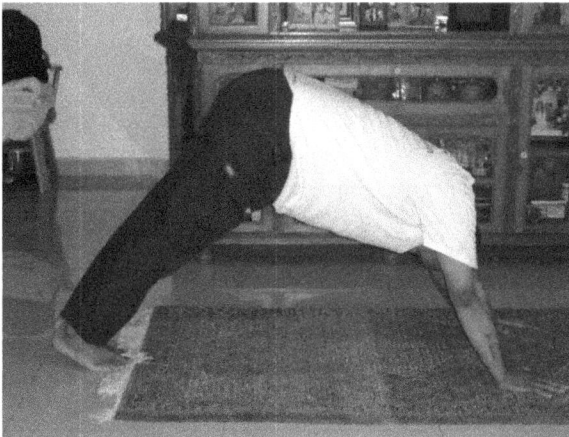

7) Now push your hips back up into the air, with your feet flat on the floor with your toes curled under onto the mat for Downward Facing Dog, an inverted posture.

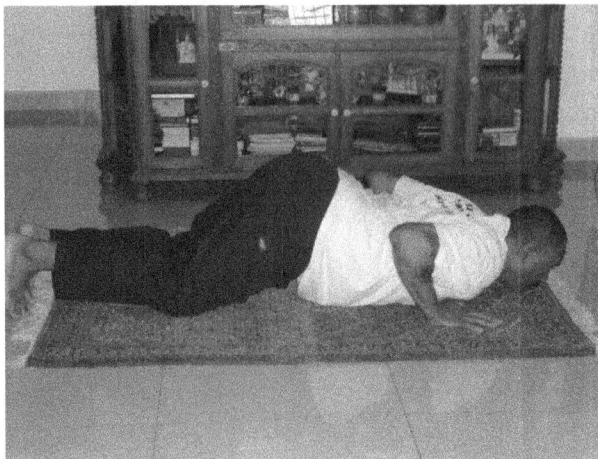

8) Come down into the Eight Limb Pose which is curled toes, your knees touch the mat, your buttocks is up, your elbows are bent and your palms are on the mat with your chest touching, your forehead or chin touches the mat.

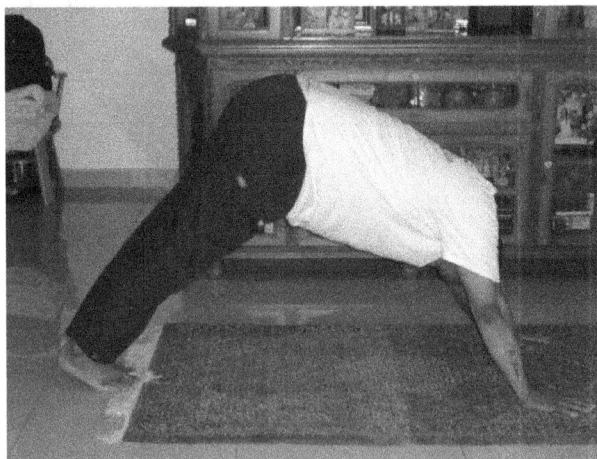

9) Move back into Down Dog and breathe in five times.

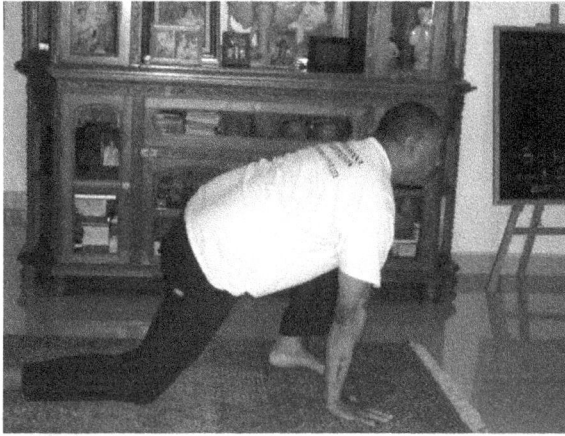

10) Bring your left leg up between your hands and get into the Lunge Pose.

Breathe in and relax, stretching your back leg and front leg at a right angle, your back is flat and your head is up. Try to pedal the feet back and forth by bending the knees to eventually get the heels on the floor. This helps to lengthen tight muscles in the back and to strengthen them. After few breaths move from "Downdog".

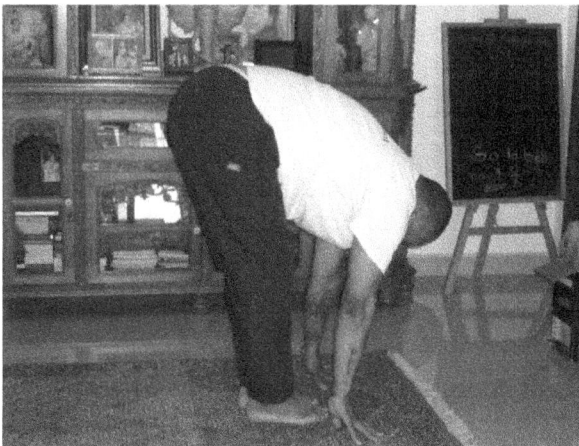

11) Bring your back leg forward to meet your front leg, with your feet together, Standing Forward Bend, in the Uttanasana pose. Lower your head, with a flat back and straight arms, place your hands beside your feet.

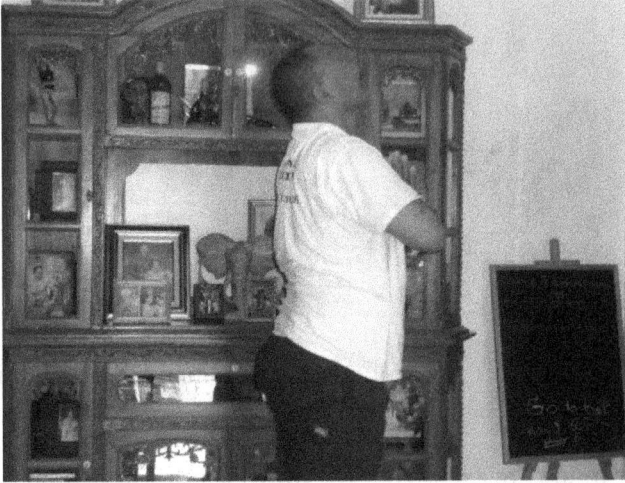

12) Breathe in and start rising slowly, one vertebrae at a time. Rise slowly and bring your hands together in Namaste' giving thanks to the ONE POWER. Come up like a ragdoll back into Tadasana as you breathe in while rising.

Standing Forward Bend Half Way - Uttiha Uttanasana

This is the half way posture of Uttanasana called Uttiha Uttanasana where your back is flat, your head comes you're your fingertips touch the floor, ankle or shins.

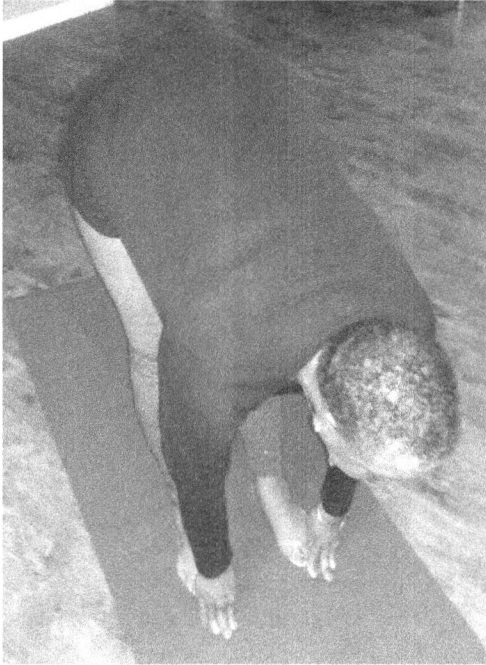

- This wakes up your hamstring and calms the mind. Legs should not be bent unless you are not quite able to do that yet.

- Keep working on it, bend, straighten, bend and straighten like pushing pedals. You should remember to breathe nice and long deep inhales through your nostrils.

Sun Salutation - Tadasana Namaste'

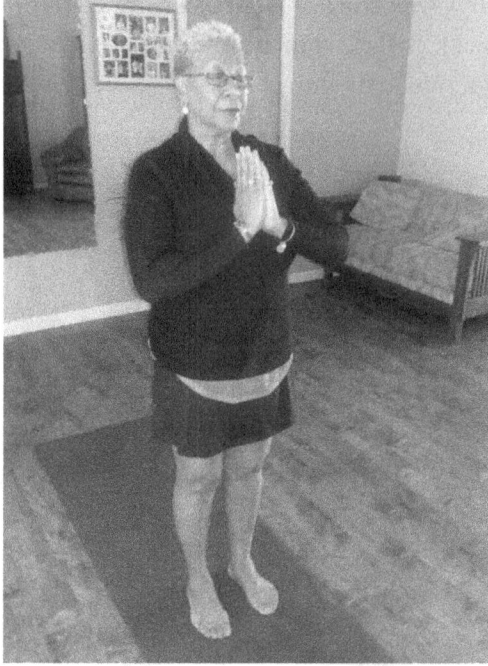

One final thought comes as spoken by Swami Muktananda - "Experience the inner silence of the thought-free state. Then the inner veil will be lifted, and the door that has been closed for so long will be opened. Suddenly the light is everywhere.

"As thoughts come up for you and as perceptions arise, be aware that they are all arising and subsiding within the ground-light of pure consciousness, the divine source. When you open your eyes and begin to look around, have the feeling that it is the light of consciousness that allows you to see and that appears in all that you see. I pray you'll be the example of divine spiritual Light to all around you. During your meditation, close your eyes and focus for a few moments on the breath."

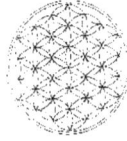

Chapter 14

A Core Practice Guide for 14 Days for You!

There are innumerable benefits in developing a strong core, torso. Your core involves the liver, gallbladder, stomach, spleen, pancreas, kidneys, adrenal glands, large and small intestines. It affects your posture and your balance and helps prevent back injury by stabilizing the pelvis.

Your core practice will utilize a combination of muscles that will leave you looking fit and feeling strong.

Here are some asanas based on the ones I teach and the variations. Spend at least fifteen minutes on a set for two weeks and watch and feel the improvement within yourself. You will feel energized, opened, and victorious and you will look fantastic!

Locust - Salabhasasna

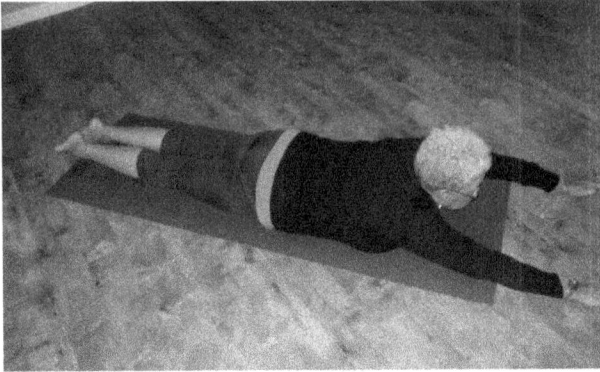

One Legged Pigeon (front & back views)
Eka Pada Rajakapotasana

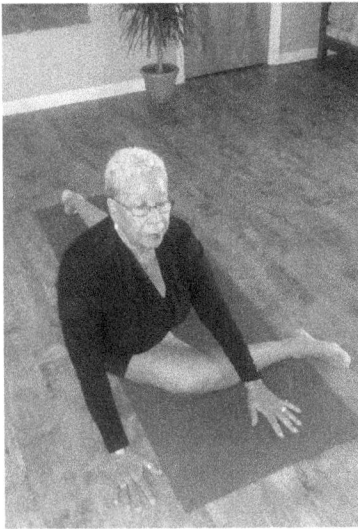

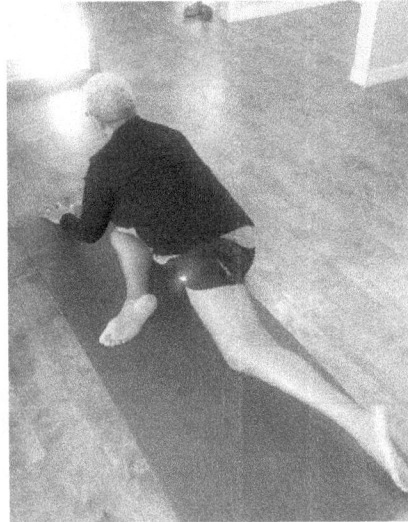

Kneel in Table Position, bring the right knee between two hands and slide the right foot next to left hand. Lay the right knee and leg at a right angle or "L" shape and press down to the floor as shown. The back leg is straightened out behind you as long and as close to the center of your mat as possible. Breathe at least five inhales and relax.

Cobbler's Pose

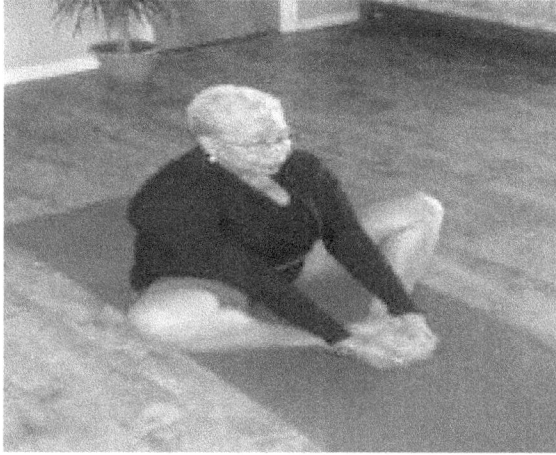

Sit with your knees bent. Open them and place the soles of your feet together. Grab your feet with both hands under and on top the feet keeping your toes touching. As you breathe in and out you will find your knees and thighs open up on their own, so muscles are being relaxed and stretched gently.

Cobra - Bhujangasana

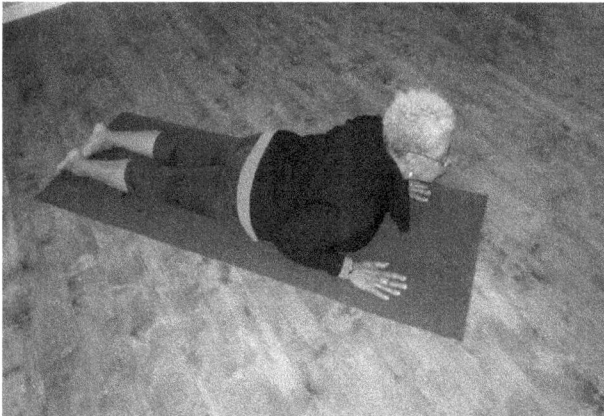

Crescent Moon Lunge Variation

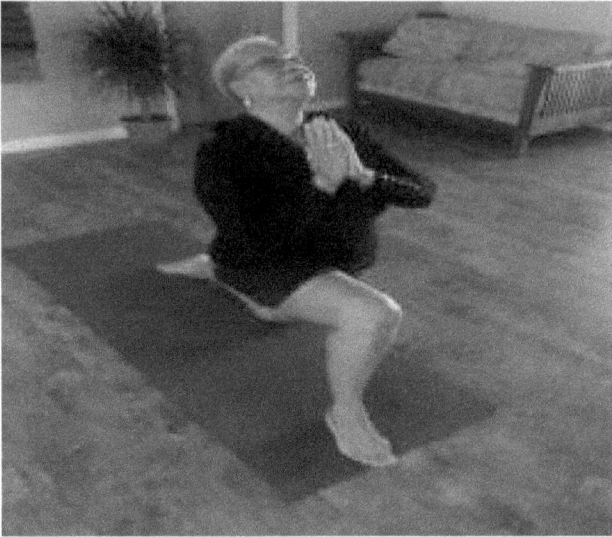

Chair Pose - Utkatasana

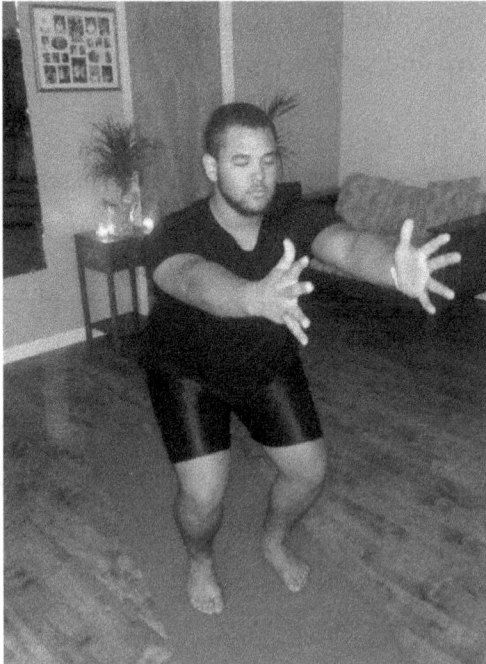

Some Standing Warm Ups:

- Arm Swings in Tadasana (4-6 times)
- Utkatasana (bend knees to ¼ squat bring arms overhead) Uttanasana (forward bend), with hands on floor look ½ way up and fold 3 times
- Bend knees, lift shoulders and come back to Tadasana (standing) or Utkatasana

Expand your horizons by moving into more challenging but still beginner poses. Namaste'.

Cow Pose - Gomukasana

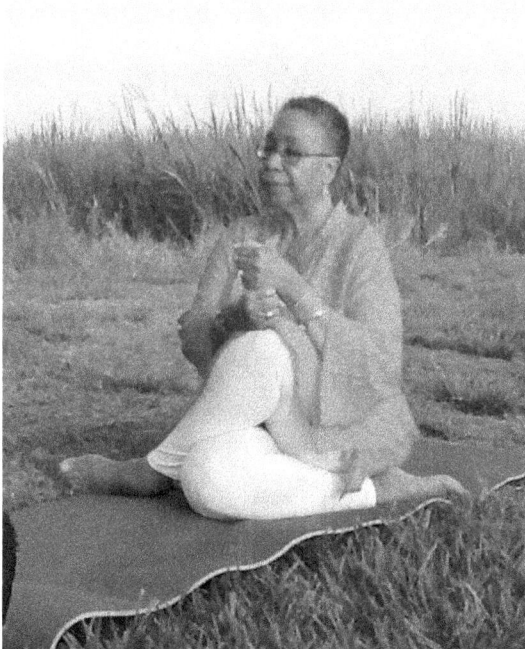

Dancer's Pose - Natarajasana

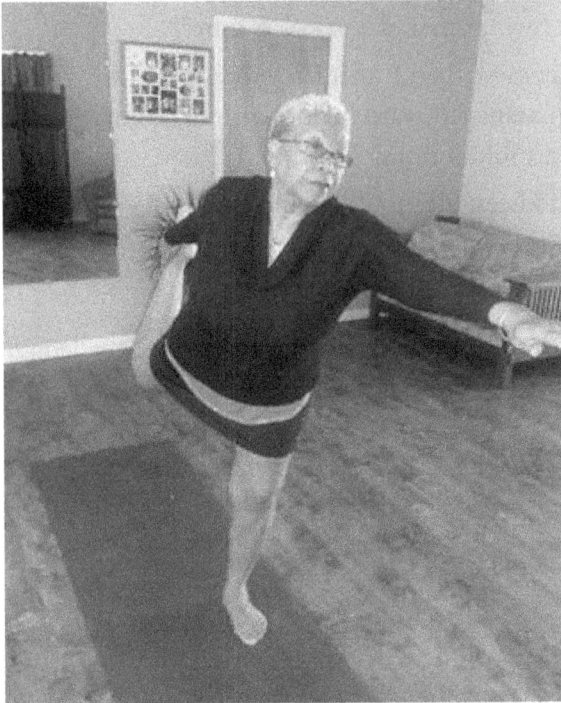

Shari Niles Boat Pose - Navasana

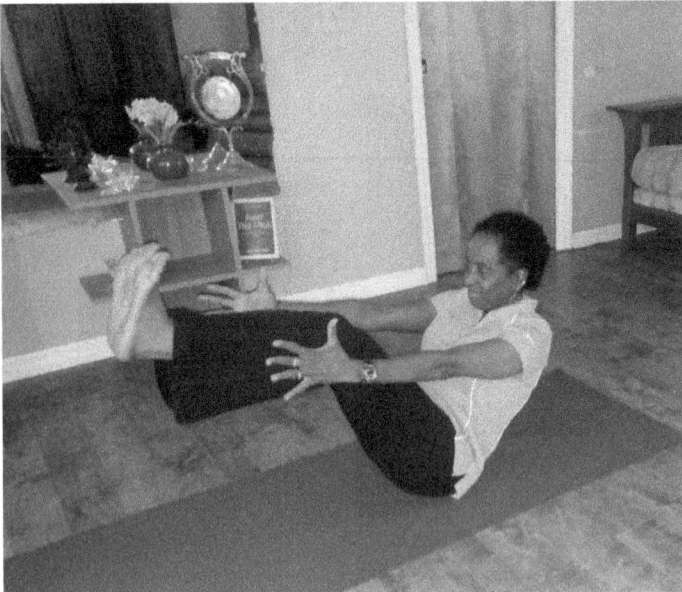

Joseph Paul Doolin Tree Pose - Vrksasana

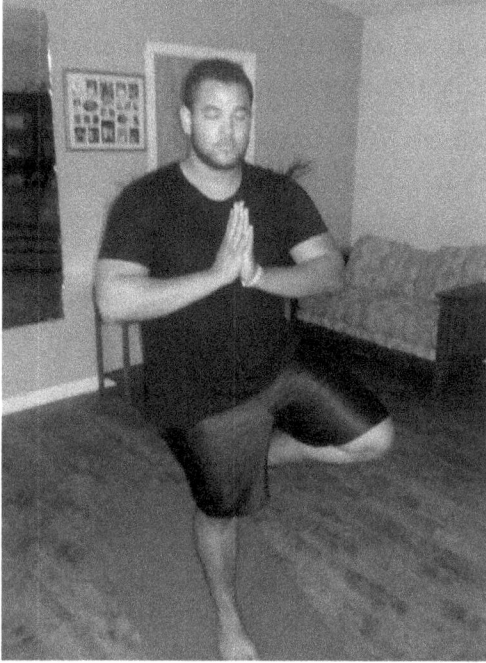

Lateral Side Angle Pose Variation - Parsvakonasana

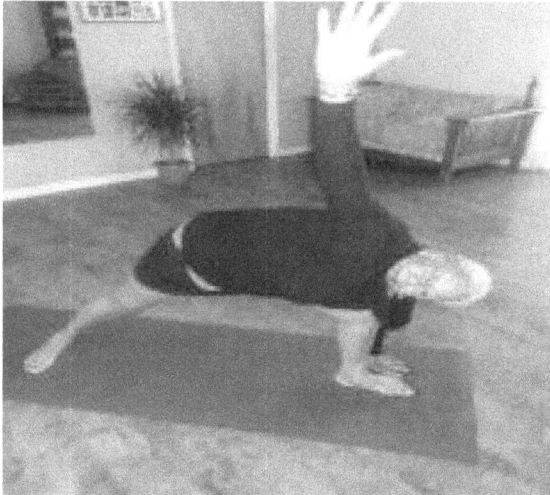

- Turn your left foot forward towards the end of the mat, while your right foot parallel to the mat. Spread you feet 3-4 feet apart.
- Lift your torso up as you inhale, bend towards your left foot, bringing the armpit of your left arm close to your bent left knee.
- Place your left palm down outside your left foot. Open your torso so you can raise your right arm up to the ceiling, with your palm open. Stack your right arm over your left arm. Breathe of course.

Yogini Daya Devi Doolin - Lateral Side Triangle

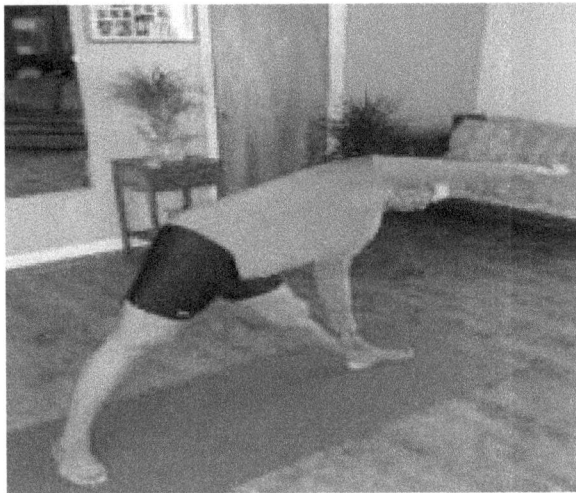

- Move from a bent left knee (Parsvokanasana) to a straightened left leg.
- Switch position of your left arm and place it in front of your left leg, with your palm firm and flat on the mat.
- Bring your right arm up and as close to your ear as possible, holding it straight, strong and firm with your breath. You can also extend your right arm so it stacks over the left arm, pointing towards the ceiling.
- Breathe in and out five times.

Rev. Daya Devi-Doolin

Internationally recognized Yoga Guru and "Thought Doctor",
Speaker and Best-Selling Author

Presents

Retreats and Workshops that nurture body,
mind and spirit

Call: (386) 532-5308
Email: padaran@padaran.com
Website: www.padaran.com

Daya Devi-Doolin offers 4 free 1 hr. packages of Gentle Hatha Yoga to VETS and PTSD VETS who sign up through www.yoga-forvets.org. She also offers yoga to domestic abused women, free upon request on the first Saturday of each month.

Recommended Bibliography

Doolin, Daya Devi, Rev. *If You Can Breathe, You CAN Do Yoga: for Beginners and the Young at Heart*; Amber Communications Group, Inc., 1334 E. Chandler Blvd., Suite 5-D67, Phoenix, AZ 85048, 2013.

Doolin, Daya Devi, Rev. *Grow Thin While You Sleep Go Figure!* Amber Communications Group, Inc., 1334 E. Chandler Blvd., Suite 5-D67, Phoenix, AZ 85048, 2013.

Doolin, Daya Devi, Rev. *The Only Way Out Is In: The Secrets of the 14 Realms to Love, Happiness and Success!* Padaran Publications, 1794 N. Acadian Drive, Deltona, FL 32725. 2009.

Doolin, Daya Devi, Rev. *Super Vita-Minds: How To Stop Saying I Hate You... To Yourself.* Padaran Publications, 1794 N. Acadian Drive, Deltona, FL 32725. 1999.

Doolin, Daya Devi, Rev. *Dabney's Handbook on a Course in Miracles.* Padaran Publications, 1794 N. Acadian Drive, Deltona, FL 32725. 1989.

Gajjar, Bharat. *Yoga for Health, Happiness & Liberation.* Sivananda Yoga Center, Wilmington, DE. 1999.

Goddard, Neville. *Your Faith is Your Fortune.* DeVorss & Co., Publishers, P. O. Box 553 Constitution Avenue, Camarillo, CA 93012-8510. 1941.

Ramacharaka, Yogi, *Fourteen Lessons in Yogi Philosophy and Oriental Occultism.* The Yoga Publication Society. Chicago 10 Illinois. 1951.

Wattles, Wallace D. *The Science of Being Great.* Top of the Mountain Publishing, 11701 Belcher Rd., S. Suite 123. Largo, FL 34643. 1983.

Yogananda, Paramahansa. *Metaphysical Meditations.* Self Realization Fellowship, 3880 San Rafael Avenue, Los Angeles, CA. 90065. 1976.

About the Author

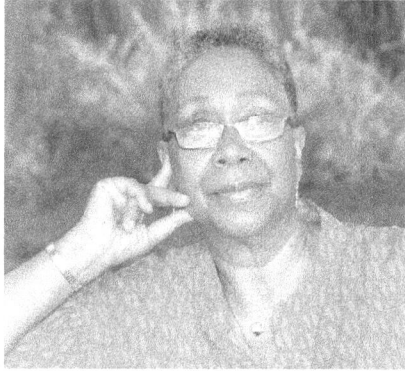

Yogini Daya Devi-Doolin is the President and Co-Owner, along with her husband Chris Doolin, of The Doolin Healing Sanctuary. She is a Registered Yoga Alliance Instructor (500).

Daya started teaching herself yoga and has been sharing her passion as an instructor for nearly fifty years. She was first trained by Professor Yogi Bharat Gajjar. She continued training and improving her skill with Yogi Amrit Desai at his Sumneytown, Pennsylvania ashram.

She continues on now with the teachings of the Sivananda Yoga Center and puts her heart and soul into teaching others. You can expect a motivating and inspiring experience when reading this book and taking a class with Daya. All of her students and you are encouraged to be positive, to leave your worries behind and to have a fun time challenging yourself to do your best. She has over a five thousand teaching hours.

She knows how important yoga has been in her life and she conveys that with all of her students so that everyone can experience the good it can bring into their lives. Yoga has transformed her body, mind and spirit and she assures you it can do the same for you as you begin to experience this journey and truth for yourself.

The Doolin Healing Sanctuary trains, teaches and offers healing of various alternatives, modalities for the mind, body and spirit. The classes that are taught, raise the vibrations of the cells to one of harmony and balancing of the chakra centers and organs. Hatha Yoga is one of the principal parts of Daya's and Chris' offerings to the community. They encourage all to stay limber, happy, healthy, fit and trim with at least one hour a day of yoga and meditation.

Other Books by Rev. Daya Devi-Doolin:

Grow Thin While You Sleep: Go Figure!

The Only Way Out Is In: The Secrets of the 14 Realms to Love, Happiness and Success!

Super Vita-Minds: How to Stop Saying I Hate You…To Yourself!

Dabney's Handbook on A Course in Miracles (with cartoons)

All I Need to Know…Is Inside (A Pocket Bite Book)

Returning to the Source (book of poems & cartoons)

Hidden Manna: How to Interpret Your Dreams

Dormck (Series of books adventures with Dabney)

Dabney, Dormck & Wiggles' Slakaduman Adventures

Dormck and the Temple of the Healing Light

Sikado's Star of Aragon (Dormck, Dabney and Wiggles' adventures)

Order Form

Telephone Orders:	602-743-7211
Email:	Amberbk@aol.com
Online orders:	WWW.AMBERBOOKS.COM

Postal Mail Orders: Send Checks & Money Orders
Payable to Amber Books
c/o Amber Communications Group, Inc
1334 East Chandler Boulevard, Suite 5-D67
Phoenix, AZ 85048

_____ copy/ies *Yoga, Meditation and Spiritual Growth for the African American Community* by Daya Devi-Doolin - $14.95

_____ copy/ies *Ageless Beauty: The Ultimage Skin Care & Makeup Book for Women & Teens of Color* by Alfred Fornay and Yvonne Rose - $15.95

_____ copy/ies *Is Modeling for You? The Handbook and Guide for the Young Aspiring Black Model* by Yvonne Rose and Tony Rose - $15.95

_____ copy/ies *Beautiful Black Hair: Real Solutions to Real Problems* by Shamboosie - $16.95

_____ copy/ies *The Afrocentric Bride: A Styling Guide* by Therez Fleetwood - $16.95

_____ copy/ies *Born Beautiful: The African American Teenagers Complete Beauty Guide* by Alfred Fornay - $14.95

_____ copy/ies *The African American Women's Guide to Successful Makeup & Skin Care* by Alfred Fornay - $16.95

Name: _____

Address: _____

City: _____ State: _____ Zip: _____

Phone: (_____)_____ Email: _____

Add $5 shipping per book
Sales tax: Add 7.05% to books shipped to Arizona addresses.

Total enclosed: $_____

Paid by:
❏ Check/Money order
❏ Credit Card #:_____ exp: _____

For Bulk Rates, Call: (602) 743-7211 or email: amberbk@aol.com

www.ingramcontent.com/pod-product-compliance
Lightning Source LLC
Chambersburg PA
CBHW072238290326
41934CB00008BB/1338